Do you have difficulty sleeping—or find that you sleep too much?

Do you have a hard time concentrating?

Do you often feel anxious and worried for "no reason?"

Are you suffering from low energy, moodiness, or crying jags?

Do you feel down or depressed?

Have you tried prescription antidepressants, but worry about their safety, or find it hard to tolerate their side effects?

If you answered "yes" to any or all of these questions, learn the secrets that people around the world have known for centuries—learn the SECRETS OF ST. JOHN'S WORT!

SECRETS of St. JOHN'S WORT

LARRY KATZENSTEIN

A Lynn Sonberg Book

St. Martin's Paperbacks

SECRETS OF ST. JOHN'S WORT

ISBN: 0-312-96574-5

Printed in the United States of America

St. Martin's Paperbacks edition/January 1998

10 9 8 7 6 5 4 3 2

To Julie, for making 1997
so memorable for us both.

A NOTE TO THE READER

This book is for informational purposes only. It is not intended to take the place of medical advice from a trained medical professional. Readers are advised to consult a physician to determine whether St. John's wort is appropriate for them before acting on any of the information or advice in this book.

Contents

CHAPTER 1

An Introduction to St. John's Wort

This book will tell you the secrets of a humble plant called St. John's wort. It's turning out to have miraculous medicinal powers—against anxiety, against insomnia and, especially, as a safe and effective treatment for mild to moderate depression. And it's fast becoming one of the biggest medical stories of the decade.

Over the past few years, you've probably heard about various herbs or other dietary supplements that have been promoted as natural remedies for depression—effective in improving mood, yet gentle to the body. Studies have shown that St. John's wort is the real thing—a natural product that lives up to its billing.

In Germany, where St. John's wort is an approved treatment for mild to moderate depression, it outsells Prozac twenty to one. Its use is also surging in other European countries. Now, the exciting news about St. John's wort has finally reached the U.S.

In the course of five months during 1997, *Time* and *Newsweek* magazines devoted feature stories to St. John's wort, *The New York Times* published two lengthy articles, and—in a segment devoted to St. John's wort—ABC's *20/20* described it as "a truly startling medical breakthrough—one that could affect millions of people who suffer from mild depression."

20/20 described St. John's wort as "an amazing herb" that is "proving to be safer, cheaper, and just as effective as prescription drugs in treating depression . . . All of us may reap the benefits."

If *you'd* like to reap those benefits, then this book can provide you with information to help you reach that goal. All you have to do is follow the three-part antidepression strategy described in the following pages:

1. HOW—AND WHY—TO GET STARTED ON ST. JOHN'S WORT

If you choose to take St. John's wort, you'll be joining millions of others around the world who already are taking the herb. The pages that follow will provide you with the information you need in deciding whether this herb is for you.

The scientific evidence—gathered through some 25 clinical studies—is impressive, and it proves that St. John's wort is not only an effective antidepressant but a remarkably safe one. In contrast, the sometimes serious side effects that can occur with standard antidepressants are alarming and well documented. If you're thinking about switching from one of these drugs to St. John's wort, a plan for doing so is mapped out within these pages. The book also describes how St. John's wort is believed to exert its antidepressant effects and what you need to know about the many types of St. John's wort products available—raw herb, teas, liquids, capsules, and tablets. All of these products are available without a prescription and are extremely safe to use, but they can vary greatly in their usefulness in improving mood. This book will tell you what the latest research says about which products are likely to be most effective, where you can get them, how long you should take them, and the proper dose for optimal benefits.

2. EAT TO BEAT DEPRESSION

More and more studies are showing that mood and food are inextricably linked. Depending on what you eat, you have the power to help defeat depression—or perpetuate it. You'll learn about the key nutrients to include in your diet that can boost your mood by elevating brain levels of the neurotransmitter serotonin. And we'll tell you which foods you should avoid—the ones that can prolong a depressed mood or even trigger a depression.

3. FOCUS ON YOUR LIFESTYLE

Stress is one of the most important factors involved in causing and prolonging depression, anxiety, and insomnia. Learn the proven tactics that can help to de-stress your life and help ward off depression. And if you are are already suffering from depression, you'll learn how to short-circuit a depressed mood and regain emotional equilibrium.

PROVEN THROUGH THE AGES

The exciting news about St. John's wort may be surprising to a lot of people, especially those who regard herbal medicine as little more than a benign but ineffective form of voodoo. But the recent findings about this herb wouldn't have surprised our ancestors; St. John's wort has been used for at least 2,500 years to treat a wide variety of ailments, ranging from snakebite to anxiety. Only in the past 20 years has the herb been rediscovered and scientifically evaluated—and re-appreciated for the many benefits it can offer. The colorful saga of St. John's wort, from an herbal remedy relied on by the ancient Greeks to a modern antidepressant used by millions, is described in

Chapter Two, "A Brief History of St. John's Wort."

This herb's most important benefit may be its usefulness against depression. The recent clinical studies on St. John's wort, carried out in Germany and other European countries, have confirmed what herbal healers have known for centuries, long before the term "depression" had even been coined: that St. John's wort helps improve the psyche by elevating mood, soothing anxiety, and helping people to think more clearly.

The clinical studies on St. John's wort have shown that this herb is not only effective in treating mild to moderate depression, but it appears to do the job as well as synthetic antidepressants. Perhaps even more important, St. John's wort is a remarkably *mild* antidepressant, one that causes far fewer of the unpleasant side effects—problems with sexual desire and performance, nausea, headache, agitation, and others—that cause many patients to abandon their antidepressant drugs. And as a bonus, St. John's wort is notably less expensive than synthetic antidepressants. St. John's wort costs about $12 a month compared with as much as $75 a month for Prozac.

MANY CAN BENEFIT

St. John's wort has the potential for improving the emotional well-being of many millions of people. That's because the herb has proven its usefulness against some of the country's most important and widespread health problems—depression, anxiety, and insomnia.

Each year, more than 12 million Americans suffer from an episode of major depression. If you're among them, and if your depression is mild to moderate in severity—the diagnosis in the majority of cases—then St. John's wort can help: clinical studies involving more than 3,000 patients have proven its effectiveness for this use.

Or you may be one of the millions of Americans with dysthymia—a chronic, mild form of depression in which people manage to function at home and on the job but are weighed down with a pessimistic outlook that makes them unable to enjoy life. If you do suffer from chronic mild depression, then St. John's wort can help you, too. In this book, when we refer to "depression," we mean either mild to moderately severe major depression or dysthymia.

Anxiety is the most common of all emotional problems—even more common than depression, and St. John's wort can help with this problem as well. In Germany, where, as mentioned, St. John's wort is an approved treatment for mild to moderate depression, it is also approved for treating anxiety.

In addition, you may also find relief with St. John's wort if you have trouble sleeping. Throughout the centuries, insomnia has been one of the main maladies for which traditional healers have prescribed St. John's wort. Studies show that the herb both improves sleep and increases alertness during waking hours.

WHAT IS DEPRESSION?

Of all the potential uses for St. John's wort, its effectiveness against depression has attracted the most interest, and for understandable reasons. Depression is a destructive, disruptive, and all-too-common health problem, afflicting about 100 million people worldwide each year. The federal government estimates that depression in the United States inflicts a severe economic burden totaling nearly $44 billion per year in health care costs, time lost from work, and other economic losses.

All of us experience the blues at one time or another—we feel down in the dumps, discouraged, pessimistic about the future. Fortunately, these feelings are usually short-lived. They last for a few hours or maybe a day or two and then we're back to being our old selves again. However, depression involves unhappiness that is both more intense and longer-lasting. In fact, depression is usually a self-perpetuating problem whose oppressive symptoms—hopelessness, fatigue, lack of energy, feelings of worthlessness or guilt—make it difficult for a person to shake off and recover from their depression, or to reach out for help.

Furthermore, it's clear that the diagnosis of depression is on the rise—the result, many experts believe, of a genuine increase in the incidence of depression. Twelve independent studies, covering

43,000 people in several different countries, have found that the rate of depression has increased during the twentieth century. While the reasons for this increase are not well understood, one possible explanation is the ever-increasing amount of stress to which people are being subjected—stress related to job insecurity, marital difficulties, balancing the obligations of work and family life, or balancing the checkbook.

Other experts point to a generational increase in depression, which appears to be unrelated to psychosocial factors such as stress. In particular, the Baby Boomers—those people born since World War II—face a greater risk of becoming depressed than people who were born before or during the war. The possible reasons for this recent surge in depression are being actively investigated and could include a genetic predisposition to depression.

Whatever the causes of today's greater prevalence of depression, the illness itself can be extremely painful, debilitating, and even fatal. About 15 percent of chronically depressed people—and 25 percent of the depressed elderly—end up commiting suicide. It's obviously important to diagnose depression so people can receive effective treatment, but that's not always easy. In fact, the difficulty in diagnosing depression is a major reason that depression is one of the most undertreated of all major illnesses, with only about one-third of its sufferers receiving treatment for their condition.

THE PROBLEMS OF DIAGNOSIS

Many depressions go undetected by the patient, his family, or even his doctor, particularly when the symptoms of depression come on gradually. Also, both patient and doctor may mistake the symptoms of depression for those of a physical illness. One study found that more than 70 percent of patients were not diagnosed by their physicians as being depressed when they should have been; as a result, these patients had to undergo numerous unnecessary tests for physical illnesses and received treatments that did nothing for their depression.

Part of the problem in diagnosing depression is that many people—including many doctors—don't understand what is meant by depressive illness. Depression actually encompasses much more than feeling depressed. In fact, it's quite possible for someone to be in the midst of a major depression without actually expressing or experiencing feelings of sadness.

For example, according to the fourth edition of the American Psychiatric Association's Diagnostic and Statistical Manual of Mental Disorders (DSM-IV), the prerequisite for being diagnosed with a major depressive episode is to have endured at least two weeks of *either* a depressed mood *or* a loss of interest and pleasure in usual activities—but not necessarily both of them. (Additionally, during the same two week period, a person must have experienced at least four other symptoms as well.)

Chapter Three ("Depression and St. John's Wort: Are You a Candidate?") discusses depression and its diagnosis in more detail. It also offers a self-test to help you determine if you're depressed and therefore might benefit from taking St. John's wort. This test, developed by the National Institute of Mental Health's Center for Epidemiologic Studies, has proven to be a sensitive tool for spotting depression. You'll also learn about the two other emotional conditions—dysthymia and anxiety—that can be alleviated by taking St. John's wort.

Fortunately, the vast majority of cases of depression can now be effectively treated, usually with a combination of psychotherapy and antidepressant medications. The antidepressants, in particular, have revolutionized the way depression is treated, and in some cases they can be lifesaving. But all of these synthetic drugs can cause bothersome and sometimes severe side effects that are often so troubling that patients stop taking them.

Chapter Four, "The Problem with Antidepressants," discusses the advantages and drawbacks of the three main types of antidepressants—the tricyclics, the monoamine oxidase inhibitors (MAOIs), and the selective serotonin reuptake inhibitors (SSRIs)—as well as the side effects associated with their use. Patients who obtain the mood-altering benefits offered by these drugs must often put up with highly unpleasant side effects. By contrast, studies show that St. John's wort causes far fewer side effects than the synthetic antidepressants—virtually none, according to some studies—while equaling their effectiveness against mild to moderate depression.

St. John's wort ranks as one of the most extensively studied of all medicinal herbs. Chapter Five, "How St. John's Wort Works Against Depression—and the Studies that Prove It," provides the latest information on how St. John's wort relieves depression while highlighting the findings of the more than two dozen clinical studies that have proven its usefulness.

The focus on St. John's wort as an antidepressant sometimes obscures the fact that it can help against other serious problems as well. Several of the herb's other important uses are described in Chapter Six, "How St. John's Wort Works Against Anxiety, Insomnia, and Seasonal Affective Disorder."

HOW TO GET STARTED

In Chapter Seven, "Your St. John's Wort Treatment Plan," you'll learn everything you need to know before you begin taking St. John's wort. You'll learn the pros and cons of all the possible forms in which St. John's wort can be taken, including tablets, capsules, teas, and liquid extracts. Discover why it's important to buy only those products that have been "standardized" to contain a guaranteed amount of hypericin, a key active ingredient in St. John's wort, and what that amount should be. This chapter also discusses the recommended doses of St. John's wort that have proven to be both effective and safe in numerous clinical trials and provides readers with information on growing and harvesting their own St. John's wort.

Finally, this chapter also offers the most comprehensive, up-to-date information available anywhere on St. John's wort products—a table listing the names of the products, where to obtain them (in health food stores or by mail order), the names, addresses, and phone numbers of the companies selling them, the form in which the products are sold (capsule, tea, etc.), how the products are standardized, and their retail prices.

ADDITIONAL ANTIDEPRESSION TOOLS

While St. John's wort works well on its own, you'll experience even better results if you include it in a comprehensive natural treatment plan that includes dietary and lifestyle changes.

Chapter Eight, "Defeating Depression Through Diet," tells you about the foods and dietary supplements that can be extremely helpful in lifting depression. For example, increasing your intake of carbohydrates can have a beneficial influence on brain levels of serotonin, the neurotransmitter that plays a key role in depression. Chapter Nine, "Coping with Depression Through Lifestyle Changes," tells why healthy and fulfilling personal relationships are so important for people with depressive illness. We'll also tell you about lifestyle measures, from meditation to stop-smoking support groups, that have proven useful in defeating depression.

Most of the publicity about St. John's Wort has centered on its ability to improve depression and other mood disorders, but the herb offers other benefits as well. For example, studies have shown that St. John's wort is a potent antibiotic, capable of killing several species of disease-causing bacteria. Researchers are hopeful that a key ingredient in St. John's wort may prove useful against HIV, the virus that causes AIDS. And in topical form, as a cream or ointment, St. John's wort has shown effectiveness in healing wounds and as an anti-inflammatory agent. Chapter Ten, "Antibiotic, Anti-inflammatory, and Other Benefits of St. John's Wort," discusses these and other possible uses of St. John's wort in more detail.

To further enlighten you about St. John's wort, answers to some of the key questions you may have about the herb can be found in Chapter Eleven, "Questions and Answers About St. John's Wort."

Finally, for those who want to learn more about either medicinal herbs or depression, we've included a chapter that lists publications, support groups, and organizations that you should know about. Chapter Twelve, "Resources," also tells you about places to go on the Internet—discussion groups, newsgroups, and other sites that anyone interested in depression, herbs, or both will find useful.

CHAPTER 2

A Brief History of St. John's Wort

St. John's wort is an aromatic perennial herb ("perennial" means that it grows season after season) that produces golden yellow flowers with five petals. It is native to Europe but now can be found growing most everywhere in the world. St. John's wort was brought to the Northeastern United States by European colonists and grows all around the country—most abundantly in California, Oregon, and Washington State.

Despite its exalted-sounding name and attractive flowers, St. John's wort is actually a rather humble plant—a weed, in fact. In California and the Northwest, it even goes by the name of Klamath weed. It is notable for being able to thrive in hostile terrain such as sandy and rocky soil and in the summer is a common sight along roadsides.

Western ranchers have been especially opposed

to St. John's wort, and they've led attempts to eradicate it from their lands, even importing an Australian flea beetle, *Chrysolina quadrigemina*, in an attempt to eradicate it. The reason: Cattle and sheep that graze on large amounts of St. John's wort can become ill due to a phototoxicity reaction, discussed in more detail in Chapter Ten. Ironically, now that the herb and its benefits have been "rediscovered," St. John's wort has been transformed from weed to cash crop, with harvesters and sellers unable to keep up with the huge demand.

POWERFUL MEDICINE

While St. John's wort may be harmful to cattle, throughout the ages and wherever it has been found, it has proven extremely useful for treating many different kinds of human maladies.

The flowering tops of St. John's wort—the flowers, unopened buds, and the upper leaves—have been ground up and used in herbal healing for more than 2,500 years. Depending on the condition being treated, the herb is either swallowed or mixed with oil and applied to the skin.

St. John's wort was known to Hippocrates who, along with being the Father of Medicine, was an authority on medicinal plants. In the first century A.D., the medicinal properties of St. John's wort were described by Dioscorides and Pliny. The former prescribed St. John's wort for sciatica, burns, and fevers, while the latter recommended mixing it with wine to treat poisonous snakebite.

HOW AN HERB GOT ITS NAME

Why the name St. John's wort? Wort is the Old English term for "plant," and the herb is named after St. John for several possible reasons. The flowers of the plant are at their most abundant around June 24, the day that the birthday of St. John the Baptist is traditionally celebrated. The name may also derive from the red spots, possibly symbolizing the blood of St. John, which appear on the flowers in August, near the anniversary of the saint's martyrdom by beheading. Finally, the plant may get its name from peoples' belief that, by placing a sprig of it under their pillow on St. John's Eve, the saint would appear to them in a dream, bless them, and protect them from death in the coming year.

Throughout St. John's wort's long history and wherever it has been used, people have believed it had supernatural powers—especially the power to chase away evil and darkness. This tradition is reflected in the plant's scientific name—*Hypericum perforatum*.

Hypericum, the genus portion of the name, is from the Greek words *hyper* (above) and *eikon* (an image or picture). This refers to the tradition of hanging the herb over pictures to ward off evil spirits and protect against demonic possession.

Because of its use in dispersing evil, one of St. John's wort's common names throughout ancient times was *Fuga Demonum*, or "Devil's Scourge."

Today, herbal experts often use the genus name *hypericum* when referring to St. John's wort. In addition, several St. John's wort products (as well as a useful site on the Internet) go by the name Hypericum. The herb's species name, *perforatum*, comes from the Latin *perforatus*, meaning perforated with small holes; this refers to the oil glands that dot the leaves as well as the petals of the plant. As it turns out, these oil glands are believed to contain some of the herb's most important medicinal ingredients.

Down through the Middle Ages, herbal texts consistently recommended St. John's wort as a useful remedy. Some of the herb's uses were cited in Gerard's *Herbal*, written around 1597, which states that St. John's wort "provoketh urine, and is right good against the stone in the bladder . . . and the leaves, flowers, and seeds stamped and put with oyle olive and set in the hot sunne, doth make an oyle the color of bloud, which is a most precious remedy for deepe wounds, and those that are thorow the body or any wound made with a venomed weapon."

In addition to being used to "provoketh urine" (i.e., as a diuretic) and for wound healing, St. John's wort was used in European folk medicine to treat bronchial inflammation, infection, hemorrhoids, burns, ulcers, and inflammation of the urogenital tract. In Russia, St. John's wort was used to treat some of these same conditions as well as gastroenteritis, rheumatism, boils, coughs, and excessive bleeding. In the United States, Native Americans have used St. John's wort for numerous purposes: the Iroquois to treat fever and as a reproductive aid; the Cherokees to treat fever, diarrhea, venereal sores and other skin lesions, to promote menstruation, and as a snakebite remedy. And—particularly pertinent for readers of this book—many societies have used St. John's wort as a "nerve tonic" for treating anxiety, fatigue, mania, and depression.

THE DECLINE OF HERBS, THE RISE OF DRUGS

Until about a hundred years ago, the world's supply of medicinal drugs consisted almost entirely of herbs. But when synthetically manufactured drugs started to appear around the end of the last century, St. John's wort and many other herbs fell into disrepute and were largely forgotten. The revival of St. John's wort began about 20 years ago in Germany, where doctors began prescribing it to their depressed patients. They noticed that most patients experienced significant improvement while suffering very few side effects. As we'll see, numerous clinical studies in recent years have confirmed the effectiveness of St. John's wort for treating depression.

In Germany, where 80 percent of physicians prescribe herbal remedies, St. John's wort products are prescribed far more often than any other antidepressant, and their popularity shows no signs of abating. Typically, German physicians turn to synthetic antidepressants only *after* St. John's wort products fail to do the job.

In 1994, 66 million daily doses of St. John's wort products were prescribed in Germany for use in treating depression. And since 1994, German sales of St. John's wort products have soared from $23 million to $71 million in 1997. For the brand known as Jarsin, German doctors write 200,000 prescriptions each month, compared with only 30,000 per month for Prozac. (In Germany, brands of St. John's wort are available both over the counter and by prescription; but about 80 percent of sales are through prescription, which allows patient to receive reimbursement from Germany's health insurance system.)

Why is St. John's wort so popular overseas yet is largely still a secret in the United States? One reason is the markedly different way that herbal medicines are regulated here compared with European countries such as Germany, where herbal medicines enjoy a status that puts them on a par with antibiotics, antihypertensives and other synthetic drugs.

In 1978, German's Federal Department of Health appointed a commission of experts, known as Commission E, to undertake a huge task: evaluate the safety and effectiveness of about 1,400 different herbal drugs derived from 600 to 700 different plant species. The commission's members were physicians, pharmacologists, pharmacists, and toxicologists, as well as representatives from consumer groups and pharmaceutical companies.

In assessing these herbal products, the commisson relied on several types of data—from animal research, human clinical trials (if such information was available), population studies, information on the historical use of herbs, the clinical impressions of physicians, the conclusions of medical associations, and the opinions of patients who had tried the herbs.

Commission E approves only those herbal medicines that it concludes are both absolutely safe and reasonably effective. Once approved by the commission, an herbal medicine can be prescribed and used like any other drug. So far, the commission has published formal reports, or monographs, on about about 300 herbs—ones that it approved, as well as ones that it didn't. These 300 herbs constitute most of the economically important herbal remedies sold in Germany.

Most herbal experts agree that the Commission E monographs contain the most thorough and scientifically valid evaluations of herbal medicines ever conducted. In the words of Dr. Varro E. Tyler, Dean Emeritus of the Purdue University School of Pharmacy and Pharmacal Sciences and one of America's most respected herb experts: "The findings of the German Commission E on herb safety and efficacy constitute the most accurate body of scientific knowledge on that subject available in the world today."

As for St. John's wort, in 1984 the commission approved it as a safe and effective antidepressant for mild to moderate cases of depression. This endorsement helped establish its legitimacy and helped propel St. John's wort to its present status as Germany's leading antidepressant of any type, natural or synthetic.

Some of the credit for the current intense interest in St. John's wort as an antidepressant belongs to Lichtwer Pharma, a German pharmaceutical company. Until a few years ago, St. John's wort was sold mainly as a bulk herb that was used to make infusions—a sort of St. John's wort "tea" that provided relatively dilute amounts of the herb's ingredients. In 1992, Lichtwer Pharma introduced the first "high-strength" St. John's wort preparation: a tablet containing 300 mg of St. John's wort extract. (An "extract" is made by soaking the chopped-up herb in a solvent such as alcohol; the solvent pulls out, or extracts, the herb's key chemicals, which remain as a powdery residue when the solvent is evaporated off. This residue contains the herb's active ingredients in a concentrated form.)

Lichtwer Pharma's high-strength product, known as Jarsin 300, was also "standardized," meaning the extract was tested and then adjusted so that it would contain a standard concentration of hypericin, one of the main active ingredients in St. John's wort. (Jarsin 300 is standardized to contain 0.3 percent hypericin.)

Today, most of the capsules and tablets on the

market also contain 300 mg of St. John's wort extract; and, like Jarsin 300, most of them—as well as many of the liquid extracts—are standardized to contain 0.3 percent hypericin. In 1997, Lichtwer Pharma began marketing Jarsin 300 in the United States under the name Kira. (More detailed information about Kira and many other St. John's wort products is available in Chapter Seven.)

BARRIERS TO ACCEPTANCE

Not only is St. John's wort accepted as an effective therapeutic drug in Germany, but it has also proven remarkably safe. Despite its extensive use in Germany, the published reports to date have not revealed serious drug interaction problems, illnesses, or deaths following overdoses. But unfortunately, the stance taken by the United States government toward St. John's wort and other herbal medicines is far less enlightened than in Germany. U.S. laws require that a product can't be marketed as a drug unless it undergoes extensive testing for safety and efficacy—testing that must include at least two clinical trials.

An herbal company in the U.S. could try to get its products approved as drugs in this way. But it's extremely expensive to do the studies required to get a new drug approved and on the market—between $300 million and $500 million. And after spending all that money, the herb company would not even have exclusive rights to its product, since herbs and other natural products can't be patented. That's the main reason there is practically no research on herbs in this country. Instead, American pharmaceutical companies ignore herbs and focus on developing synthetic drugs with unique formulas that are patentable.

This legal situation prevents useful herbs such as St. John's wort from being marketed as the drugs they truly are. Instead, they're sold in health food stores, pharmacies, and supermarkets as dietary supplements. And if the label of an herbal product states that the herb is effective for some condition—a statement regarded as a drug claim—the FDA can seize the product or take legal action against its producer for marketing an unapproved new drug. So when you examine the labels on St. John's wort and other herbal products, you'll see that they're largely devoid of information about what the herb can do for you.

When drug companies have shown interest in medicinal plants, they have focused on finding—and then patenting—the ingredient considered mainly responsible for the plant's therapeutic effect. They may then extract the key chemical from the plant or devise a way to make large amounts of the chemical synthetically.

Drugs produced in this way can certainly be useful—as shown by Taxol, the breast cancer drug derived from the bark of the Pacific yew tree, and approved in 1993 for treating advanced breast and ovarian cancers. But focusing on a single chemical in an herb overlooks the possible benefits offered by the entire herb. With St. John's wort and many others, medicinal effectiveness probably stems not from any single ingredient but from several chemicals acting in concert to produce the desired therapeutic benefit.

St. John's wort, for example, contains at least 40 different chemicals belonging to several different chemical classes. One of these 40 chemicals— hypericin—had been thought to be mainly responsible for St. John's wort's antidepressant effects. (As we'll see, this is the reason that St. John's wort products are usually "standardized" to contain a certain percentage of hypericin by weight). But recent studies suggest that the antidepressant effect produced by St. John's wort comes from beneficial changes in several different chemical pathways in the brain—which almost certainly is due to the action of several of the herb's chemicals rather than just one.

Over the past 10 years, as European interest in St. John's wort has surged, experts there have extracted the herb's chemicals and attempted to find how each may be contributing to St. John's wort's many medicinal benefits. The table at the end of this chapter lists 10 of the chemicals or chemical classes extracted from St. John's wort that appear to be bioactive, and it summarizes their possible therapeutic effects.

THE HERBAL ADVANTAGE

Herbs have given the world some of its most important medicines—quinine, derived from the bark of the cinchona tree, for treating malaria; reserpine, from the roots of the tropical shrub rauwolfia, for high blood pressure; digitalis, from the foxglove plant, for relieving the pain of angina; and vincrisitine and vinblastine, the alkaloids from the periwinkle plant that are used for treating lymphomas and other types of cancer. In fact, an estimated one-fourth of all drugs now in use have been derived from plant sources.

Herbs can be thought of as dilute drugs containing one or more "bioactive" (meaning that have a physiological effect) ingredients. But perhaps the best definition of an herb is the one coined by Dr. Varro E. Tyler, the American herb expert cited earlier. Tyler defines herbs as "crude drugs of vegetable origin utilized for the treatment of disease states, often of a chronic nature, or to attain or maintain a condition of improved health."

Clearly, *herbal* medicine—consuming the many chemicals that an herb has to offer—can provide benefits that individual, isolated chemicals may not offer. In the case of St. John's wort, this multiplicity of chemicals has been found to produce an antidepressant effect equal to that of the single-ingredient antidepressants, but with a much gentler impact on the body and far fewer side effects.

If you're looking for a treatment that will lift your mood, but that is also extremely safe and inexpensive, then St. John's wort may be the answer you've been seeking. And this book can be your guide for using it wisely and well.

Table 1
The Activity of Certain Constituents of St. John's wort

Constituent	Activity
Amentoflavone (13', 118-biapigenin)	Anti-inflammatory, useful in healing ulcers
GABA (gamma-aminobutyric acid)	Sedative effect
Hyperforin	Antibacterial against gram-positive bacteria; wound-healing; alters levels of neurotransmitters; potential use in cancer treatment
Hypericin	Antiviral, potential use in cancer treatment
13,118-biapigenin	Probably sedative
2-methyl-butenol	Sedative
Proanthocyanidins	Antioxidant, antibacterial, antiviral, vasodilator (relaxes blood vessels)
Pseudohypericin	Antiviral
Quercitrin	Antidepressant effect
Xanthones	Antidepressant effect, antibacterial, antiviral, diuretic, improves heart function

Adapted from *St. John's Wort: Quality Control, Analytical and Therapeutic Monograph.* American Herbal Pharmaco-poeia, July 1997.

❧ CHAPTER 3 ❧

Depression and St. John's Wort: Are You a Candidate?

You can be sure that St. John's wort is causing the pharmaceutical companies considerable anxiety. Antidepressants are among the most lucrative of all drugs for these companies, yet St. John's wort offers what many people would prefer: a natural, effective, and much less expensive way to improve mood and restore tranquility.

Are you a candidate for the many benefits that St. John's wort has to offer? This chapter will help you decide. It tells you what you need to know about depression—what causes it, who is most susceptible, and how the problem is diagnosed. It also offers a self-test so that you can assess whether you might be depressed and whether you should consider taking St. John's wort or some other treatment. Finally, it offers some recommendations regarding the safe use of St. John's wort.

A HEAVY TOLL

Depression, the problem that probably affects most users of St. John's wort, is an illness that must be taken seriously. In some form, depression affects 25 percent of all women, 10 percent of all men, and five percent of all adolescents world-wide. In the United States, it is one of the most common of all psychological problems, afflicting more than 12 million people each year. It can cause extreme emotional pain and leave its sufferers unable to function, contemplating suicide and, all too often, committing it. An estimated 15 percent of untreated or inadequately treated depressives eventually commit suicide; and among suicide victims, more than half are suffering from a depressive illness.

The good news about depression is that it can usually be successfully treated with antidepressant drugs, psychotherapy or a combination of the two. And the exciting news about St. John's wort is that it appears to work as well as antidepressant drugs in treating mild to moderate depression while causing far fewer side effects.

NOT A SIGN OF WEAKNESS

When we talk about "depression" in this book, we're referring to what used to be called "clinical depression" and is now generally termed "major depression"—a serious illness that robs life of all pleasure and can make getting through the day all but impossible.

Despite being so widespread and potentially fatal, major depression is all too often ignored or not recognized for what it is, either by the person suffering from it or his or her doctor. Alternatively, the physical symptoms of depression—sleep problems, fatigue, or weight loss, for example—may be mistaken for some other illness, resulting in treatment that does nothing to help the depression. Unfortunately, relatively few victims of depression get the help they need and too many people suffer needlessly—never realizing that their fatigue and chronic irritability may be symptoms of an underlying depression. Surveys done in communities indicate that fewer than half of all people who suffer from major depression are ever treated.

Episodes of depression typically last for six months and then clear up, even if no treatment is given. Some people experience only a single episode of major depression during their lifetimes. But major depression more commonly is a recurrent disorder: More than half of patients who have one depressive episode will experience others later in life. Effective treatment, including the use of antidepressant medications, can help cut short the pain and anguish of a depressive episode. And putting patients on maintenance doses of medication can help to prevent later depressive episodes from occurring.

Many people are afraid even to contemplate the idea that they might be suffering from depression because they view depression as a sign of emotional weakness—as something that they should be able to "pull themselves out of" if only they had enough will power. But while researchers still don't know the precise cause or causes of depression, recent insights indicate that depression is primarily a biochemical problem. It involves an imbalance of chemicals in the same way that Type I diabetes is caused by a lack of insulin. A person can't be expected to "pull himself out of" a major depression any more than a diabetic can be expected to maintain proper blood sugar levels without insulin.

A depressed mood can be one of the most painful events that a person can suffer in life. And, unfortunately, the stigma of being perceived as mentally ill prevents many people with depression from seeking the help they need. If you are depressed, you owe it to yourself, your family, and your friends to do something about it, since you *can* overcome it.

Major depression appears to result from an imbalance of the brain's neurotransmitters—chemicals, such as serotonin and dopamine, whose actions are responsible for our moods. Today's antidepressants, including Prozac, Paxil, Serzone, and St. John's wort, work to treat depression by restoring the proper levels of one or more of these neurotransmitters.

In some cases, depression can occur out of the

blue, for no apparent reason. But in other cases, depression's biochemical imbalances can be triggered by external events—an acute or chronic physical illness, certain prescription drugs, excessive alcohol consumption, or traumatic or stressful life events such as divorce, the death of a loved one, loss of a job, or a move to a new city.

THE SYMPTOMS OF DEPRESSION

Why do some people bounce back from these traumas, while others fall into a depression? People are susceptible to depression not because they're emotionally weak or fragile but, in most cases, because they inherit a predisposition to depression.

Researchers have shown that if one identical twin suffers from depression, there is a 70 to 80 percent chance that the other twin will also be affected. But among *nonidentical* twins in which one twin is depressed, there is only about a 15 percent chance that his twin will also be depressed—about the same risk that *any* depressed person's close relatives (other siblings, parents, or children, for example) will be depressed. More distant relatives of a depressed person—grandparents, uncles, or aunts—have about a seven percent risk. And the risk that a person with no family history of depression will become depressed is only about two to three percent. This diminished risk of depression with decreasing genetic similarity supports the idea that genetics may play a significant role in depression.

Depressive illness shouldn't be confused with the temporary emotional ups and downs that everyone experiences—the periods of sadness brought about by unhappy events that can include everything from the loss of a job to a loss by our hometown football team. Depressive illness should also not be confused with the intense grief that occurs when someone close to us has died. These feelings of sadness and grief are normal and temporary reactions to the vicissitudes of life. In most cases, time successfully heals those wounds, our dark feelings abate, and we return to functioning normally.

By contrast, people with major depression don't bounce back from the blues. They remain disturbed for months and sometimes even years. Their illness affects their feelings, thoughts, behaviors, and their body.

When deciding whether a patient is depressed, psychiatrists and other mental health professionals rely on the American Psychiatric Association's Diagnostic and Statistical Manual (DSM). The latest edition, the fourth, is referred to as DSM-IV. To be diagnosed as suffering from major depression, DSM-IV requires that a person must display five or more of nine possible symptoms for at least two weeks. At least one of the symptoms must be either

- Depressed mood for most of the day, nearly every day

or

* Markedly diminished interest or pleasure in all, or almost all, activities most of the day, nearly every day (as indicated either by the patient's subjective account or by others who observe that the patient is apathetic most of the time)

The other seven possible symptoms are:

* Significant weight loss when not dieting, weight gain, or decrease or increase in appetite nearly every day
* Insomnia or excessive sleepiness nearly every day
* Observable restlessness or lethargy nearly every day
* Fatigue or loss of energy nearly every day
* Feelings of worthlessness or excessive inappropriate guilt nearly every day
* Diminished ability to think or concentrate, or indecisiveness, nearly every day
* Recurrent thoughts of death, recurrent thoughts of suicide without a specific plan, a suicide attempt, or formulating a specific plan for committing suicide

Mental health professionals gauge the severity of a patient's depression according to how many of the nine possible symptoms the person has and how intensely the patient is experiencing them. Studies have shown that people with major depressions of mild to moderate severity can benefit from St. John's wort.

ARE YOU DYSTHYMIC?

Even if you are not suffering from major depression, St. John's wort could also help you if you're one of the millions of Americans with dysthymia—a milder but chronic form of depression.

Over the years, dysthymia has gone by different names—"depressive neurosis" in the 1950's and "depressive personality" in the 1970's. Dysthymia usually begins in childhood or adolescence and often persists for years or even decades—so long, in fact, that people who have this mood disorder often don't recognize that they're depressed but instead regard their gloomy mindset as part of their personality.

Dysthymia can be thought of as sort of an emotional tapeworm that saps a person's ability to function at maximum capacity, enjoy life, or feel good. Instead, people with dysthymia "endure" life and never really feel well. They go through the motions of living with no real enthusiasm while perpetually feeling down in the dumps—pessimistic, discouraged, and hopeless.

The symptoms of dysthymia are basically the same as for major depression—you just don't need as many to qualify, and they're generally not as intense or severe. While a diagnosis of depression requires the presence of five or more of the DSM-IV symptoms (listed above) over a two-week period, a diagnosis of this milder form of depression requires the presence of two or more of these symptoms for at least two years (one year for children or adolescents).

Despite their depressed mood, people with dysthymia can often continue to function at a very high level. They don't experience their disorder as a depression but instead are affected in other ways. They may feel irritable all the time or have such low self-esteem that, even when they walk into a party where they have many friends, for example, they assume that people don't like them.

Since people with dysthymia typically don't think of themselves as ill, it's not surprising that they usually don't seek help for their problem. They've felt hopeless about life for so long that they believe "That's just the way I am." But fortunately, the cloud of dysthymia can be lifted. The synthetic antidepressants such as Prozac can do the job, but so can St. John's wort—and with far fewer unpleasant side effects.

Some people with dysthymia also experience episodes of major depression, with their symptoms becoming dramatically more severe for awhile and then returning to their usual muted level. These people are said to have "double depression"—dysthymia plus major depression.

Both major depression and dysthymia appear to be caused by the same basic problem: an imbalance of serotonin and other neurotransmitters in the brain. St. John's wort, by gently bringing these chemicals back into balance, can help in treating both of these depressive conditions.

TEST YOUR OWN DEPRESSION LEVEL

If you want to assess your own level of depression, you can take a widely used test known as the CES-D (Center for Epidemiological Studies—Depression), which was developed by Lenore Radloff at the National Institute of Mental Health. For the following 20 items, simply circle the choice that best describes how you have felt over the past week:

1. **I was bothered by things that usually don't bother me.**
   0 Rarely or none of the time (less than 1 day)
   1 Some or a little of the time (1-2 days)
   2 Occasionally or a moderate amount of the time (3-4 days)
   3 Most or all of the time (5-7 days)

2. **I did not feel like eating; my appetite was poor.**
   0 Rarely or none of the time (less than 1 day)
   1 Some or a little of the time (1-2 days)
   2 Occasionally or a moderate amount of the time (3-4 days)
   3 Most or all of the time (5-7 days)

3. **I felt that I could not shake off the blues even with help from my family and friends.**
   - 0 Rarely or none of the time (less than 1 day)
   - 1 Some or a little of the time (1-2 days)
   - 2 Occasionally or a moderate amount of the time (3-4 days)
   - 3 Most or all of the time (5-7 days)

4. **I felt that I was not as good as other people**
   - 0 Rarely or none of the time (less than 1 day)
   - 1 Some or a little of the time (1-2 days)
   - 2 Occasionally or a moderate amount of the time (3-4 days)
   - 3 Most or all of the time (5-7 days)

5. **I had trouble keeping my mind on what I was doing.**
   - 0 Rarely or none of the time (less than 1 day)
   - 1 Some or a little of the time (1-2 days)
   - 2 Occasionally or a moderate amount of the time (3-4 days)
   - 3 Most or all of the time (5-7 days)

6. **I felt depressed.**
   - 0 Rarely or none of the time (less than 1 day)
   - 1 Some or a little of the time (1-2 days)
   - 2 Occasionally or a moderate amount of the time (3-4 days)
   - 3 Most or all of the time (5-7 days)

7. **I felt that everything I did was an effort.**
   - 0 Rarely or none of the time (less than 1 day)

1 Some or a little of the time (1-2 days)
2 Occasionally or a moderate amount of the time (3-4 days)
3 Most or all of the time (5-7 days)

8. I felt hopeless about the future.
0 Rarely or none of the time (less than 1 day)
1 Some or a little of the time (1-2 days)
2 Occasionally or a moderate amount of the time (3-4 days)
3 Most or all of the time (5-7 days)

9. I thought my life had been a failure.
0 Rarely or none of the time (less than 1 day)
1 Some or a little of the time (1-2 days)
2 Occasionally or a moderate amount of the time (3-4 days)
3 Most or all of the time (5-7 days)

10. I felt fearful.
0 Rarely or none of the time (less than 1 day)
1 Some or a little of the time (1-2 days)
2 Occasionally or a moderate amount of the time (3-4 days)
3 Most or all of the time (5-7 days)

11. My sleep was restless.
0 Rarely or none of the time (less than 1 day)
1 Some or a little of the time (1-2 days)
2 Occasionally or a moderate amount of the time (3-4 days)
3 Most or all of the time (5-7 days)

12. I was unhappy.

    0 Rarely or none of the time (less than 1 day)
    1 Some or a little of the time (1-2 days)
    2 Occasionally or a moderate amount of the time (3-4 days)
    3 Most or all of the time (5-7 days)

13. I talked less than usual.

    0 Rarely or none of the time (less than 1 day)
    1 Some or a little of the time (1-2 days)
    2 Occasionally or a moderate amount of the time (3-4 days)
    3 Most or all of the time (5-7 days)

14. I felt lonely.

    0 Rarely or none of the time (less than 1 day)
    1 Some or a little of the time (1-2 days)
    2 Occasionally or a moderate amount of the time (3-4 days)
    3 Most or all of the time (5-7 days)

15. People were unfriendly.

    0 Rarely or none of the time (less than 1 day)
    1 Some or a little of the time (1-2 days)
    2 Occasionally or a moderate amount of the time (3-4 days)
    3 Most or all of the time (5-7 days)

16. I did not enjoy life.

    0 Rarely or none of the time (less than 1 day)
    1 Some or a little of the time (1-2 days)

    2 Occasionally or a moderate amount of the
       time (3-4 days)
    3 Most or all of the time (5-7 days)

17. I had crying spells.
    0 Rarely or none of the time (less than 1 day)
    1 Some or a little of the time (1-2 days)
    2 Occasionally or a moderate amount of the
       time (3-4 days)
    3 Most or all of the time (5-7 days)

18. I felt sad.
    0 Rarely or none of the time (less than 1 day)
    1 Some or a little of the time (1-2 days)
    2 Occasionally or a moderate amount of the
       time (3-4 days)
    3 Most or all of the time (5-7 days)

19. I felt that people disliked me.
    0 Rarely or none of the time (less than 1 day)
    1 Some or a little of the time (1-2 days)
    2 Occasionally or a moderate amount of the
       time (3-4 days)
    3 Most or all of the time (5-7 days)

20. I could not get "going."
    0 Rarely or none of the time (less than 1 day)
    1 Some or a little of the time (1-2 days)
    2 Occasionally or a moderate amount of the
       time (3-4 days)
    3 Most or all of the time (5-7 days)

To tally your score, just add up all the numbers that you have circled. The higher your score, the greater the degree of your mood disturbance. A score of 22 or higher indicates that you may be suffering from an episode of major depression. A somewhat lower score—perhaps on the order of 15 to 21—could mean that you are suffering from dysthymia.

TAKE CARE BEFORE SELF-TREATING

From what you've read so far in this chapter and from taking this self-test, you may have concluded that you suffer from depression or dysthymia. If you have, then you may indeed be a candidate for St. John's wort. But just as diabetics shouldn't prescribe insulin for themselves, you shouldn't embark on therapy with St. John's wort on your own. Instead, you should first consult a health care professional, for several reasons.

The main reason for a professional consultation is that *depression is not something to be taken lightly*. As we've noted, depression can render people virtually unable to function and can lead to suicide when it's untreated or inadequately treated.

Deciding that you may be depressed and that you may benefit from a treatment such as St. John's wort is the crucial first step on the road to relief from your symptoms. But if you *do* think you may be suffering from major depression or dysthymia, you should get your self-diagnosis confirmed by someone with expertise in mental illness—perhaps your family doctor, but preferably a mental health expert such as a psychiatrist or clinical psychologist.

A mental health expert can assess your mental state by doing a rigorous examination—the only way to determine reliably whether you're depressed or not. If you are depressed, the expert may conclude that St. John's wort really isn't the best treatment for you—perhaps because your depression is too severe or because you're suffering from some other problem entirely. Above all, if you have thoughts of suicide or feel overwhelmed by your depression, put this book down and seek help without delay!

Again, St. John's wort has been proven effective in treating mild to moderate depression. But studies to show whether it helps relieve severe depression simply haven't been performed. People who are severely depressed may have hallucinations or attempt suicide. They may require Prozac or one of the other synthetic antidepressants proven effective against more severe forms of depression, and they may even need to be hospitalized. Similarly, there is no evidence that St. John's wort can help people who have serious psychiatric problems such as biopolar disorder (manic-depressive illness) or schizophrenia.

IT'S NOT FOR EVERYBODY

Many people believe that because a substance such as St. John's wort is "natural," it must therefore be perfectly safe. St. John's wort certainly is much less likely to cause unpleasant side effects than one of the synthetic antidepressants. Considering the fact that millions of Europeans have been taking it over the past decade, this herb has proven remarkably safe, with very few reports of any problems.

Nevertheless, the many clinical studies involving St. John's wort clearly show that it is a drug (and before taking any drug, it's a good idea to consult your physician). St. John's wort acts on the body to relieve depression, probably by altering levels of those neurotransmitters in the brain that govern mood. Actually, St. John's wort should probably be thought of as a "multidrug," since it contains a dozen or more different chemicals that are "bioactive," and recent studies suggest that the herb relieves depression by altering the levels of not one but several of the brain's neurotransmitters.

Since St. John's wort is a drug, there is always the possibility of side effects. But luckily, in the case of St. John's wort, those side effects are almost always minor and very infrequent. To minimize the risk of side effects, though, certain people should not take St. John's wort, and the herb should be avoided in the following situations:

• *Don't take St. John's wort if you're pregnant.* It's a standard recommendation to pregnant women. To avoid possible harm to the fetus, try to minimize your exposure to all drugs during your pregnancy, especially during the first trimester. That warning should also include St. John's wort, which clearly functions as a drug when swallowed. But for those women who might be taking St. John's wort while not aware that they're pregnant, what is known about St. John's wort's possible toxicity is reassuring.

In 1996, researchers published the results of toxicology studies in which rats and dogs were fed very high amounts of a St. John's wort extract for six months. No effects were observed on the animals' fertility or reproduction. In addition, there was no evidence that St. John's wort has the potential to cause mutations in cells.

• *Children and nursing women should not take St. John's wort.* When nursing women are taking drugs, a trace of the drug often ends up in their milk. Since babies can't effectively metabolize certain drugs, it's possible—although highly unlikely—that St. John's wort could be toxic for them. Since the herb's safety when taken by babies and children has not been studied, it's a good idea to err on the side of caution.

• *If you have fair skin, try to minimize your exposure to the sun if you take St. John's wort.* Hypericin, a compound found almost exclusively in St. John's wort, can cause photosensitivity reactions (mainly skin reddening) in people who consume St. John's wort products and are then exposed to sunlight. Until recently, such photosensitivity reactions were thought to be limited to cattle and sheep that grazed on large quantities of St. John's wort; it was assumed that people consuming the much lower amounts found in St. John's wort extracts didn't have to worry. But a study published in 1996 found that the extracts could cause mild photosensitivity problems in people as well.

This study involved volunteers who took Jarsin 300, Germany's best-selling St. John's wort extract. For 15 days, the volunteers took twice the recommended dose (i.e., they took 600 mg three times daily, rather than the normal 300 mg three times a day) and were also exposed to UV-A radiation (long-wave ultraviolet light, the kind involved in triggering photosensitivity reactions).

These volunteers experienced some erythema (increased skin redness) from the combination of St. John's wort and UV exposure. This skin redness was mild and transient, disappearing a few days after St. John's wort was discontinued. No other adverse effect was noted in this study, even though volunteers used twice the recommended dose.

If you have fair skin don't exceed the recommended dose of St. John's wort and minimize your exposure to the sun. (As we'll see in Chapter Ten, researchers are taking advantage of hypericin's photosensitizing properties and have achieved promising results when using this chemical as a cancer treatment.)

• *Don't take St. John's wort while you're also taking Nardil, Parnate, or other members of a class of antidepressants called monoamine oxidase inhibitors (MAOIs).* One of the ways St. John's wort may alleviate depression is by acting the way Prozac does, i.e., as a selective serotonin reuptake inhibitor, or SSRI. (We discuss Prozac's action in more detail in Chapter Four, "The Problem with Antidepressants.") Serious and even fatal reactions, including hyperthermia and coma, have occurred when people have taken Prozac in combination with one of the MAOIs. Since St. John's wort may have Prozac-like actions, the standard recommendation made for Prozac should apply to St. John's wort as well: Don't take it in combination with an MAOI or within 14 days of discontinuing therapy with an MAOI.

And since St. John's wort *may also* act as a MAOI, the converse situation should also apply—meaning it's probably not a good idea to take St. John's wort if you're also taking Prozac or one of the other SSRIs. This is to avoid the same sort of serious reactions, mentioned above, that can occur when MAOIs and SSRIs are taken together.

Until recently, it was assumed that St. John's wort's antidepressant ability was entirely due to its MAOI activity. Recent studies in animals have failed to find that it affects this enzyme, and experts now believe that St. John's wort produces its antidepressant effect through other biochemical pathways. Nevertheless, the possibility that St. John's wort may have *some* MAOI activity cannot yet be completely ruled out. So, to be on the safe side, you probably shouldn't take St. John's wort if you're also taking an SSR1 such as Prozac, Paxil, or Zoloft.

• *People taking illicit drugs or narcotics (heroin, cocaine, crack, or speed, for example) shouldn't take St. John's wort.* Such drugs could produce dangerous interactions when taken with St. John's wort. And some of these drugs can actually contribute to depression.

St. John's wort is especially appropriate for mild cases of anxiety and for mild to moderate depression—the kind that most affected people have. If this is your problem, then St. John's wort should work as well as the synthetic antidepressants in making you feel better, while at the same time causing virtually no side effects. Your doctor may well agree that St. John's wort can help you. If so, Chapter Seven, "Your St. John's Wort Treatment Plan," can help you choose products that are suitable for you and also help you to select the proper dose.

CHAPTER 4

The Problem with Antidepressants

While synthetic antidepressants have revolutionized the way depression is treated, they share a major drawback: All of them can cause side effects—including ejaculatory difficulties and other sexual problems—that may be so severe that significant numbers of patients stop taking them. By contrast, St. John's wort appears to be equally effective in treating mild to moderate depression, yet is not known to cause sexual difficulties or, for that matter, *any* serious side effects.

This chapter will describe the side effects associated with the three major classes of synthetic depressants—the monoamine oxidase inhibitors (MAOIs), the tricyclics, and the newest products, the selective serotonin reuptake inhibitors (SSRIs), which include Prozac, Paxil, and Zoloft. But first we'll note three important advantages that St. John's wort has over *all* of the synthetic antidepressant drugs.

Freedom from sexual side effects. All antidepressants can cause sexual problems including impotence, reduced sexual desire, delayed or absence of orgasm, and delayed or painful ejaculation—some of the main reasons that patients stop taking these drugs. Prozac, the best-selling antidepressant, causes reduced sexual desire, delayed orgasm, and other sexual effects in up to 75 percent of men who take it; in women, the drug may reduce sexual desire. Yet Prozac is far from alone in causing these side effects. In fact, many other antidepressant drugs—especially the MAOIs and the tricyclics—are much more likely to cause sexual problems than Prozac is.

Just why sexual side effects occur with these antidepressant drugs isn't clear, but it probably has to do with the fact that all of them alleviate depression by altering neurotransmitter levels in the brain. Such changes alter brain pathways that affect mood, but they also affect other pathways as well, including those involved in sexual arousal and performance.

In contrast to the frequent sexual side effects from synthetic antidepressants, St. John's wort is notable for causing scarcely any. The two dozen clinical studies involving St. John's wort contain no reports of sexual problems of any kind. Just how St. John's wort works to relieve depression isn't known. But however it does the job, St. John's wort has the distinction of doing it without interfering with patients' sex lives.

Especially suited to elderly patients. Depression in older people can be a serious problem—particularly because the depressed elderly are more likely to commit suicide than younger people. (People over 75 make up about twelve percent of the population but account for seventeen percent of all suicides.) But unfortunately, prescribing antidepressants for the elderly can be a complicated business. Antidepressants are less well tolerated in the elderly; and because so many of them are taking medications for other health problems, the risk of drug interactions may be signficiant. For these reasons, St. John's wort may be an especially appropriate treatment for depressed older people.

In 1994, the *Journal of Geriatric Psychiatry and Neurology* published a special issue devoted entirely to studies on St. John's wort. In introducing these studies, the journal's editor noted that "one of the most important features [of St. John's wort] is that side effects are rarely observed. Allergic reactions occur rarely. This benign side effect profile may make [St. John's wort] a particularly attractive choice for treating mild to moderate depression in our elderly patients."

No interactions with alcohol. People taking antidepressants are frequently warned to avoid alcohol, particularly if they drive, because of the risk of drowsiness and auto accidents. But St. John's wort does not appear to interact with alcohol. In a 1993 study, 32 healthy male and female volunteers took either a St. John's wort extract or a placebo in combination with alcohol; they were then given a series of cognitive and psychomotor tests, including a test of driving skill. In this small study, no differences were observed between the St. John's wort group and the placebo group, suggesting that alcohol might not interact with St. John's wort. Nevertheless, it's probably a good idea to err on the side of caution and not mix the two.

THE BENEFITS OF ANTIDEPRESSANTS

Their side effects notwithstanding, synthetic antidepressants—in use now for 40 years—have helped many thousands of people and probably have saved many lives as well, by preventing suicide. People whose depressions could previously be alleviated only by drastic means such as electroconvulsive therapy can now experience improved mood after just a few weeks of treatment. In general, about two-thirds of people who are depressed will respond to any given antidepressant. And even if people don't respond to the first antidepressant they try, they have an excellent chance of receiving help from another of the many effective synthetic antidepressant drugs now on the market.

As one of their main benefits, antidepressants can interrupt the all-too-common self-sustaining spiral of depression—when a depressed mood causes the person to withdraw from pleasurable activities and social support, which in turn deepens the depression and causes the person to withdraw even more. And by elevating mood, antidepressants help a person become more engaged in life again. Ideally, people are rid of their depression after several weeks or months of treatment and later can cope with life without the need for drugs.

For many people, antidepressant drugs have literally been lifesavers. For many others, these drugs or a combination of drugs and psychotherapy has allowed them to continue functioning— holding down jobs and caring for families. But as helpful as they are for millions of people, antidepressants have a serious downside as well.

SIDE EFFECTS CAN BE SEVERE

All synthetic antidepressants cause side effects that can range from merely unpleasant to potentially life-threatening. Many people find these side effects so intolerable that they abandon antidepressants, only to see their depression recur. For people troubled by their antidepressants but who nevertheless continue taking them, these side effects can seriously erode their quality of life, leaving them feeling chronically drugged, tired, or dizzy—or with other persistent problems such as dry mouth, impotence, headache, or abdominal distress.

THE MAOIS: EFFECTIVE BUT SOMETIMES FATAL

Monoamine oxidase inhibitors (MAOIs) are synthetic drugs that prevent the enzyme monoamine oxidase from breaking down three neurotransmitters—norepinephrine, serotonin, and dopamine—and therefore cause the levels of all three to increase in the synapses, the gaps between nerve cells in the brain. The two most frequently prescribed MAOIs, phenelzine (Nardil) and tranylcypromine (Parnate), are both effective in treating major depression.

But unfortunately, the MAOIs can cause significant side effects—rapid heartbeat, sedation, dizziness, insomnia, sexual problems (including inability to obtain an erection), constipation, and agitation. But most important in terms of the risks associated with the MAOIs, a potentially fatal hypertensive reaction can occur if a person taking a MAOI antidepressant also consumes aged cheese or other foods containing high amounts of the amino acid tyramine.

The enzyme monoamine oxidase, present in the lining of the intestinal tract and liver as well as in the brain, normally breaks down tyramine so that very little gets into the bloodstream. But if someone taking a MAOI antidepressant eats a food rich in tyramine, the amino acid isn't broken down but instead is absorbed into the bloodstream. Tyramine then gets into the cells of the body and triggers the release of norephinephrine, which can cause a rapid rise in blood pressure. This "cheese reaction" can cause severe headaches, flushing, profuse perspiration, blurred vision, vomiting, and even death from intracranial hemorrhage.

Not surprisingly, people taking a MAOI antidepressant must adhere to a strict diet that excludes not only cheese but also other tyramine-rich foods including fermented meats, chicken liver, fava or broad beans, overripe bananas, sherry, brandy and red wines (especially Chianti), beer, yogurt, sour cream, raisins, and avocados. Finally, in order to avoid a dangerous episode of high blood pressure, people taking MAOIs must avoid a number of prescription and over-the-counter drugs that have stimulant properties, including nasal decongestants, diet pills, and numerous cold, allergy, sinus, asthma, and hay fever medications.

Most books and articles about St. John's wort warn that people taking the herb for depression or any other reason should adhere to the same dietary and drug restrictions required for patients on MAOIs. The reason: It has long been thought that St. John's wort relieves depression by functioning as an MAOI. Recent studies in animals, however, have failed to find such a monoamine oxidase-inhbiting effect.

As we explain more fully in Chapter Five, "How St. John's Wort Works Against Depression," the current thinking is that if St. John's wort does block monoamine oxidase, the inhibition must be extremely mild. As a result, experts now believe that people taking St. John's wort probably don't need to be so restrictive about the foods they eat and the drugs they take.

Another side effect of MAOIs is also relevant to users of St. John's wort. Studies indicate that the effects of MAOIs on the brain persist for four weeks or more after treatment ceases. If a patient begins taking Prozac or another SSRI while a MAOI is still present in the body, a hypertensive reaction can occur that has proven fatal to several people who've taken both types of antidepressant at the same time.

Since St. John's wort was thought to function as a MAOI, people have usually been warned against taking the herb if they're also taking Prozac or another SSRI. As we noted on page 47, that precaution is worth following. But because St. John's wort does not appear to act as a MAOI, the danger of such interactions appears to be slight. For example, millions of Europeans have taken St. John's wort over the past 10 years—and, according to experts, at least several hundred of them have taken St. John's wort and Prozac (or one of the other SSRIs) at the same time. To date, published reports have not cited a single case of an adverse effect attributed to consuming St. John's wort and an SSRI simultaneously. *For that matter, we know of no published reports of drug interactions between St. John's wort and any other drug.*

THE TRICYCLICS: PLENTY OF UNPLEASANT EFFECTS

Tricyclic antidepressants were the most commonly used antidepressants for 30 years—from the late 1950's, when they were first marketed until the late 1980's, when a new type of antidepressant—SSRIs—took over, beginning with Prozac in 1988. Over those three decades, millions of depressed people took tricyclic drugs with names like Tofranil, Elavil, Sinequan, and Anafranil. (The term "tricyclic" refers to the molecular structure of these drugs.)

Tricyclics produced excellent results—and in fact, their 70 percent success rate in treating depressed patients remains unsurpassed by any other antidepressants new or old. But many people who took tricyclics were plagued with side effects that ranged from the merely annoying to downright disabling.

The tricyclics, like SSRIs, inhibit nerve cells in the brain from "reuptaking" neurotransmitters. But rather than being selective in the neurotransmitters they affected, the tricyclics increased brain levels of several of them, particularly serotonin and norepinephrine. This impact on more than one neurotransmitter may help explain why tricyclics are potent drugs, but it probably also accounts for the many nasty side effects that these drugs cause.

Dry mouth is one of the most common of the side effects caused by tricyclic antidepressants. These drugs may also dry out the eyes, making it diffucult for people to wear contact lenses, and they can also cause blurred vision and a worsening of glaucoma in people who already have this eye disease. Tricyclics generally cause the heart to speed up by 20 or more beats per minute—which can be an annoyance if your heart is healthy, but can be downright fatal if you have heart disease.

Tricyclic antidepressants also tend to lower blood pressure—especially in older people, who may feel dizzy when standing up or climbing out of bed and who then may fall and break a hip. Other significant side effects include constipation, reduced urine flow, fatigue, increased weight gain (as much as 30 pounds in some cases), sexual problems (including impotence, loss of sexual interest and inability to ejaculate), and risk of suicide (the tricyclics are the leading cause of death by drug overdose in the United States).

Most insidious of all, tricyclics can make users feel as though they're functioning in a perpetual mental fog. People often become acclimated to this effect or assume that it's a part of their depression; but once they stop taking the drug, they immediately notice the improvement in their mental acuity.

The tricyclics are excellent antidepressants, but as a practical matter the people taking them often don't fare well, since they often have to lower their prescribed dosage in order to avoid side effects. In one study of more than 2,000 depressed outpatients taking tricyclics, fewer than one-third of patients actually took the recommended dosage of their drug. In view of all the adverse side effects associated with tricyclics, it's no surprise that they've now been largely superseded by SSRIs—which, while not as toxic as the tricyclics, are still far from perfect.

THE SSRIS: MANY PROBLEMS REMAIN

Prozac, the first of the new class of SSRI antidepressants, was first marketed in January 1988. It has since been joined by several other SSRIs including Zoloft, Paxil, Serzone, and Luvox. If the tricyclics can be thought of as acting as biochemical "shotguns," affecting several different neurotransmitters, then the SSRIs are more like rifles, aimed at raising levels of just one neurotransmitter, serotonin.

When Prozac ushered in the era of the SSRIs, it was hoped that these drugs would be just as effective as the tricyclics but would cause fewer side effects, thanks to their singularity of action. And to some extent, those hopes have been realized. Studies comparing Prozac and other SSRIs with older antidepressants show that SSRIs appear equally effective, even when it comes to treating cases of severe depression. And since SSRIs do cause fewer side effects than the older drugs, patients are better able to tolerate them. SSRIs are being used not only to treat depression but for other emotional problems such as obsessive-compulsive disorder, panic attacks, eating disorders, and PMS.

All of the SSRIs differ slightly in the side effects they cause and how long it takes them to "kick in" (patients typically don't begin to notice the effects until after they've been taking any SSRI for two to four weeks). But all of these drugs act on the brain in the same basic way: by affecting the brain levels of an important neurotransmitter known as serotonin.

TARGETING SEROTONIN

The brain's billions of nerve cells communicate with each other largely via neurotransmitters. Typically, a nerve cell, or neuron, will manufacture a neurotransmitter and then excrete it into the gap, or synapse, between it and an adjoining nerve cell. When the neurotransmitter makes contact with a receptor on the surface of the second nerve cell, the "message" or nerve impulse is then transmitted from one nerve cell to the next. Millions of such messages are sent every second in the human brain.

So far, several dozen of these chemical messengers, or neurotransmitters, have been identified. Several of these neurotransmitters—norepinephrine, dopamine, and serotonin—seem to play major roles in governing a person's mood; and all the antidepressants (the MAOIs, tricycylics, and SSRIs) work by boosting brain levels of one or more of these chemicals.

Among the mood-affecting neurotransmitters, serotonin seems to be especially important. It's the primary neurotranmsitter that drug designers have targeted over the past 10 years in trying to synthesize antidepressant drugs—an effort that has led to the development of Prozac and the other SSRIs now on the market.

All the SSRIs are based on the notion that depression often results from abnormally low levels of serotonin in the gaps, or synapses, between the nerve cells. The SSRIs boost synaptic levels of serotonin, and this increase serves to rev up communication among nerve cells and eventually results in improved mood.

The SSRIs increase serotonin levels between the cells by capitalizing on the fact that the nerve cells, or neurons, are frugal when it comes to their neurotransmitters and do their best to recycle them. Shortly after neuron A communicates with adjacent neuron B by releasing a dose of serotonin molecules into the synapse between the two cells, neuron A will reabsorb these serotonin molecules through use of special receptors on its surface known as reuptake pumps. Prozac and all the other SSRIs somehow block these pumps so that serotonin can't be reabsorbed by neuron A. The result: reuptake of serotonin is selectively blocked, serotonin molecules accumulate in the synapses— and depressions are lifted.

DOES PROZAC PROVOKE VIOLENCE?

Since the SSRIs work as well as the older anti-depressants while causing fewer side effects, they've become the most popular class of antidepressants. Prozac in particular is a phenomenal success story—it is by far the most widely prescribed psychiatric drug in history. In 1996 alone, 20 million prescriptions were written for the drug. But Prozac has also proven extremely controversial, with some critics charging that the drug should never have been approved.

One of the most serious criticisms of Prozac is that it can trigger suicidal and violent behavior in people who take it. National interest in such a link was sparked by a 1989 incident in Louisville, Kentucky, in which a man went on a shooting rampage, killing eight people and wounding a dozen others before taking his own life. An autopsy showed that the man had been taking Prozac.

The concern over suicide due to Prozac arose the following year. It was prompted in large part by a paper, "Emergence of Intense Suicidal Preoccupation During Fluoxetine [Prozac] Treatment," that was published in the February 1990 issue of the *American Journal of Psychiatry* and written by Dr. Martin Teicher of Harvard Medical School. Teicher stated that "six depressed patients free of recent suicidal ideation developed intense, violent, suicidal preoccupation after two to seven weeks of fluoxetine [Prozac] treatment." Two of these patients tried unsuccessfully to kill themselves. The suicidal thinking of all the patients disappeared when Prozac was discontinued.

Teicher's report aroused intense media interest in Prozac's possible dark side and prompted dozens of lawsuits against the drug's manufacturer, Eli Lilly & Co. Most of these suits charged that the drug was unsafe and that the company had failed to inform physicians that Prozac could lead to suicidal or violent behavior.

It turned out, however, that Teicher's study may have unfairly indicted Prozac as the cause of the suicidal attempts and thoughts. Four of the six patients were taking medications in addition to Prozac that may have been responsible, and five of the patients suffered from other serious health problems including alcoholism, bulimia, and manic depression. And while none of the patients may have had "recent" suicidal thoughts, all six patients had had suicidal tendencies before taking Prozac—they'd either thought about committing suicide or had attempted it at some point in their lives.

Despite these flaws in the Teicher report, it did prompt experts to look closely at clinical studies involving Prozac to see whether the patients taking Prozac are at greater risk of commiting suicide or a violent act than people not on the drug. For the most part, the findings have been reassuring.

For example, 18 separate clinical trials were recently analyzed in which Prozac was studied for its effectiveness in treating a variety of problems other than depression. In these trials, which involved about 4,000 patients, all the documented aggressive behaviors were four times more common among patients taking placebos than among patients on Prozac.

It appears that Prozac is no more likely than other antidepressants to trigger suicidal tendencies in patients. It does appear possible, however, that Prozac and other synthetic antidepressants can cause sudden suicidal behavior in a small minority of depressed people. One possible explanation: A small number of people are so depressed that, even though they've thought about committing suicide, they lack the energy required to follow through and actually perform the act. But after they've taken an antidepressant for a few weeks, the drug's energizing effect—an effect common to all synthetic antidepressants, not just Prozac—gives these people the strength to act on their suicidal impulses.

Unfortunately, this energizing effect of synthetic antidepressants usually kicks in before the drugs' mood-enhancing effects have a chance to take hold. As a result, for potentially suicidal people who take synthetic antidepressants, there may be a "window of vulnerability"—the first two to six weeks after they've begun therapy, when these people are experiencing the energizing effects of the drugs but have not yet obtained their mood-elevating benefits.

In contrast to the possible risk of suicide posed

by synthetic antidepressants, St. John's wort appears to have a much better record of safety in this regard. Millions of depressed people have taken hundreds of millions of doses of St. John's wort over the years, and although there have been no formal studies of a possible link between St. John's wort and suicide, there have been no published reports of suicide attributed to taking the herb.

Moreover, some synthetic antidepressants—particularly the MAOIs—pose a risk to patients with suicidal tendencies because overdoses of these drugs can prove fatal. But with St. John's wort, overdoses seem to have little effect. There has not been a single published case report of harm due to someone taking an overdose of the herb.

OTHER PROZAC PROBLEMS

Although Prozac should be acquitted on the most serious charge against it—that it causes suicide and violent behavior—the drug is nevertheless open to criticism on several other counts. One of the most outspoken critics of Prozac is Dr. Peter Breggin, who outlined the case against the drug in his book *Talking Back to Prozac*. In arguing that Prozac is ineffective, unsafe, and should be taken off the market, Breggin makes the following points that have particular relevance when it comes to assessing the safety and effectiveness of St. John's wort:

- *Surprisingly few patients were actually tested*

on Prozac prior to the drug's approval by the FDA.

Before the FDA approves a psychiataric drug, it requires that the drug's manufacturer carry out two or more research protocols—each usually encompassing several studies—to demonstrate that the drug is safe and effective. These studies typically involve hundreds or even thousands of patients. But according to Breggin, in Prozac's case the actual number of patients receiving Prozac was actually much smaller than implied by its manufacturer, Eli Lilly & Co.

In a letter it sent to doctors, Eli Lilly & Co. stated that "more than 11,000 individuals participated in clinical trials for Prozac, including over 6,000 treated with Prozac." But according to Breggin, most of these patients apparently were not enrolled in placebo-controlled trials—the only type of study considered relevant for learning if a drug is effective. Breggin used the Freedom of Information Act to obtain the raw data on the Prozac studies from the FDA. He found that the FDA had concluded that only three of the research protocols, involving 17 studies, were adequate from a scientific standpoint to use as evidence for approving Prozac.

Breggin went through each of the 17 studies and added up the the number of Prozac patients who actually completed the four-, five- or six-week trials that the FDA used as the basis for approving Prozac. "The grand total," he writes, "turned out to be a meager 286 patients." He concludes that it is "safe to guess that few if any physicians or patients who rely on FDA studies have any idea that the actual number of Prozac patients completing the trials was so small."

These findings are particularly relevant when it comes to St. John's wort. As we'll see in the next chapter, a study published last year in the *British Medical Journal* analyzed 23 clinical trials in which St. John's wort had been compared with either a placebo or a standard synthetic antidepressant. The authors of this study concluded that these 23 trials—in which more than 1,700 patients participated—showed that St. John's wort was significantly more effective than a placebo in treating depression and that it may work as well as standard antidepressants.

Indeed, if Prozac was actually tested on fewer than 300 patients, then the clinical evidence for St. John's wort's effectiveness against depression is stronger than that supporting the usefulness of Prozac.

• *In almost all cases, the clinical studies carried out to gain FDA approval of Prozac lasted only a few weeks.*

Most people assume that, in the clinical studies done to gain a drug's approval, the patients take the drug for months or even years. But the clinical studies carried out on Prozac generally lasted for just five or six weeks. According to Breggin, "Eighty-six percent of all the patients in all the studies were treated for three months or less. Only 63 patients took Prozac for more than two years before completion of the premarketing studies and the FDA approval of Prozac." Breggin concludes that "in effect, anyone now taking Prozac for more than a few weeks is part of a giant ongoing experiment on its longer-term effects."

Breggin may have a point here—at least when it comes to possible long-term adverse effects from taking Prozac. But from all indications, an antidepressant's effectiveness can be established by relatively short-term studies such as these. Clearly, in approving Prozac, the FDA considered five- and six-week clinical trials as being of sufficient length to show that this drug was able to alleviate depression in patients.

But ironically, the effectiveness of St. John's wort in treating depression was recently questioned because clinical trials on it lasted "only" about the same amount of time. In an editorial accompanying the *British Medical Journal* study cited above, the authors complained: "Of the four trials that have compared a hypericum [St. John's wort] preparation with a synthetic antidepressant, none lasted longer than six weeks."

Here we have an example of the double standard applied to "standard" drugs and medicinal herbs. What has long been recognized as an acceptable length of time for a trial of a synthetic antidepressant is considered too brief a study to show that an herb such as St. John's wort is effective.

PROZAC AND SEXUAL PROBLEMS

In addition to Breggin's criticisms, there is ample evidence that Prozac—although it causes significantly fewer adverse reactions than the MAOIs or the tricyclic antidepressants—is by no means free of causing side effects. In fact, it's not uncommon for such side effects to cause people to abandon the drug.

Following is a discussion of the most important side effects associated with Prozac. Where appropriate, we note other SSRI drugs that are also known to cause the same adverse effects and what is known about the role of St. John's wort in causing these problems.

Sexual problems. One of the initial attractions of Prozac as an antidepressant was that it supposedly did not interfere with sexual performance, sexual sensation, or sexual interest. Indeed, the studies carried out to gain FDA approval of Prozac indicated that sexual problems rarely afflicted patients taking the drug.

The results from these studies, summarized in the *Physicians Desk Reference*, indicate that only 1.6 percent of patients experienced decreased libido and 1.9 pecent experienced sexual dysfunction. But soon after Prozac came on the market, studies started to appear indicating that sexual problems due to Prozac were much more common than had earlier been reported.

For example, in a study published in 1993 in the *Journal of Clinical Psychiatry*, a physician reported on his findings after questioning 60 of his male patients about problems they'd experienced while taking Prozac. He found that 75 percent of these patients reported they either had difficulty ejaculating during sex or were unable to do so. Lowering the dose of Prozac helped to ease the problem, and it disappeared when the men stopped taking the drug.

In yet another study, also appearing in 1993 in the *Journal of Clinical Psychiatry*, a team of researchers came to this conclusion: "While the manufacturer's information indicates that sexual dysfunction associated with the serotonin-selective reuptake inhibitor fluoxetine [Prozac] occurs in less than two percent of patients, recent reports suggest the incidence may be much higher ([from] 7.8 percent to [a] 75 percent incidence of male sexual dysfunction)."

Why did sexual problems rarely show up in the studies carried out before Prozac was approved? One possible explanation is that there was no requirement that patients in these early studies be questioned about drug-induced sexual difficulties. And unless people are asked about personal and potentially embarrassing issues of this sort, they usually don't provide such information.

Disturbances in sexual functioning have now turned out to be the main problem associated with the SSRIs in general and Prozac in particular. (Such problems have caused many people to stop taking the drugs, putting them at risk for a recurrence of their depression.) For men, these problems include failure to achieve orgasm, painful orgasms, or (less commonly) failure to obtain an erection. For both men and women, the sexual problems associated with Prozac include decrease or absence of sexual desire and delayed orgasm. Current estimates are that nearly half of patients can expect to experience some sort of sexual problem from taking Prozac.

Two of the more recently approved SSRIs, Paxil and Zoloft, are also notable for their high rates of sexual problems—primarily ejaculatory difficulty—experienced by men who take these drugs. In the clinical trials of Paxil, nearly 13 percent of men had ejaculatory difficulties, primarily ejaculatory delay, and 10 percent had other sexual problems, including impotence and the inability to achieve an orgasm. Among women taking Paxil, nearly two percent had difficulty reaching orgasm. In the Zoloft trials, nearly 16 percent of men reportedly had sexual difficulties, primarily ejaculatory delay, while nearly two percent of women experienced problems. If the same discrepancies between clinical findings and real-life experience hold true for these drugs as they did with Prozac, then the true incidence of sexual problems associated with Paxil and Zoloft is likely to be much higher than the percentages noted here.

By contrast, St. John's wort's effect on sexual desire or sexual function appears to be minimal—and most likely nonexistent. Some two dozen clinical studies involving St. John's wort have been carried out, without a single report of a sexual problem that has been experienced by someone taking the herb. (Two new synthetic antidepressants, Serzone and Wellbutrin, are also notable for rarely causing sexual side effects. These drugs are not classified as SSRIs; and in fact, as with St. John's wort, it's not clear just how these two drugs act to alleviate depression.)

Stimulant effect. For significant numbers of people who take it, Prozac appears to have a stimulant effect that causes anxiety and various other types of agitation. For example, the *Physicians Desk Reference* states that, based on clinical trials involving Prozac, 14.9 percent of patients reported nervousness while on the drug, 9.4 percent reported anxiety and 7.9 percent experienced tremors. Unfortunately, lowering the dose of Prozac usually doesn't help.

But while Prozac *causes* anxiety in nearly 10 percent of patients, St. John's wort has been approved in Germany for *treating* anxiety. In its Commission E monograph on St. John's wort (discussed in more detail in Chapter Two), the German government's list of approved uses for St. John's wort includes, in addition to depression, "anxiety and/or nervous unrest."

Insomnia. Depressed people are often troubled by insomnia. They often have trouble falling asleep, or they wake up very early in the morning—or they may experience both problems. So it's not good to take an antidepressant that con-

```
955          10    5754   02142  002

RX 0177998        1N      3.00
ST JOHN WORT      1T      5.99
NEWSPAPERS        1N       .35
     SUBTOTAL             9.34

  7% SALES TAX            .42
  TOTAL                  9.76

    CASH     9.76 CHANGE        .00

          THANK YOU
  JANUARY 14, 1998      1:24 PM
```

Items purchased at Walgreens
may be returned to any of our
stores within 30 days of
purchase.

Items with a receipt will be
exchanged, refunded in or
credited to your account.

Items without a receipt will be
exchanged or refunded in mail
within 14 days.

For any refund you may be
asked for acceptable
identification

JANUARY 14, 1998   1:24 PM

tributes to insomnia—yet Prozac causes insomnia in a signifcant proportion of patients, particularly in the early weeks of treatment. In general, about 15 percent of patients can expect to experience insomnia after starting on Prozac.

The other SSRI antidepressants, such as Paxil and Zoloft, also have the potential for causing sleep disturbance. Among all the synthetic antidepressants currently available, the one least likely to disrupt sleep appears to be Serzone. This drug rarely disturbs sleeping and seems, if anything, to help correct sleep disturbances in depressed patients. In this respect, Serzone ranks with St. John's wort, which is notable for not disrupting the sleep of people who take it. And, as described more fully in Chapter Six, "How St. John's Wort Works Against Anxiety, Insomnia and Seasonal Affective Disorder," research indicates that St. John's wort may improve the quality of sleep by causing an increase in slow-wave sleep during two of the deep stages of sleep.

Drowsiness. Although numerous people experience agitation while taking Prozac, Paxil, or other SSRIs, many others experience the contrary effect of drowsiness. An estimated one in five people taking Prozac or other SSRIs feel drugged or drowsy while on the drugs, and about five percent of people stop using such drugs because of that side effect. In some cases, this drowsiness is a result of the insomnia that these drugs cause. By contrast, St. John's wort does not cause drowsiness and may actually help to improve alertness.

Headache. Many people who are depressed experience headache as a symptom of their depression. Unfortunately, Prozac and other SSRIs may cause tension or migraine headaches or make them worse. Prozac causes headaches in about 20 percent of patients using it, while St. John's wort is not known to cause headaches.

Digestive system problems. Thirteen percent of people taking Prozac experience a reduced appetite and subsequently lose a significant amount of weight—an effect that usually occurs at the beginning of treatment and that, unfortunately for those who want to shed some pounds, usually doesn't continue. In fact, significant numbers of people who take Prozac find that they gain weight while on the drug. Other digestive system effects caused by Prozac include nausea (affecting 21.1 percent of patients), diarrhea (12.3 percent affected), dry mouth (9.5 percent), indigestion (6.4 percent), abdominal pain (3.4 percent), and vomiting (2.4 percent). St. John's wort has also been known to cause cases of gastrointestinal upset, but they occur much less frequently than with Prozac.

Other problems. Prozac also causes a number of other side effects that range from merely irritating to serious. These include excessive sweating (affecting 8.4 percent of patients) as well as skin rashes, abnormal dreams, and seizures (affecting 0.2% of patients). The only one of these problems attributed to St. John's wort is skin rash, which may occur when fair-skinned people taking the herb are exposed to sunlight.

Prozac and the other SSRIs are definitely better tolerated than the earlier classes of antidepressants, the MAOIs and tricyclics. But as we've seen, they're far from perfect, and they cause side effects in a significant percentage of people who take them.

ST. JOHN'S WORT SIDE EFFECTS: FEW AND MILD

By contrast, the extensive clinical experience with St. John's wort indicates that it appears to equal the synthetic antidepressants in effectiveness while causing far fewer side effects: While about one-fourth of Prozac users can be expected to experience one or more distressing side effects, studies show that fewer than 10 percent of patients experience side effects with St. John's wort and these effects are almost always quite mild.

In 1996, a study in the *British Medical Journal* looked at side effects in clinical trials involving St. John's wort. In six trials in which it was compared with a standard antidepressant, only 0.8 percent of patients being treated with St. John's wort dropped out because of side effects compared with three percent of patients treated with a standard antidepressant. And the herb even did well when matched against a placebo. In 13 placebo-controlled trials, 4.1 percent of patients on St. John's wort experienced side effects versus 4.8 of patients treated with a placebo; and only 0.4 percent of St. John's wort patients dropped out due to side effects compared with 1.6 percent of patients on placebo.

The safety of St. John's wort has also been demonstrated through drug monitoring studies, in which patients taking a drug are closely observed by their doctors in order to collect information on a drug's side effects as well as its effectiveness. Perhaps the most extensive such study was published in Germany in 1993. This drug-monitoring study involved 3,250 depressed patients, all of whom were treated for four weeks with an extract of the herb. The average age of the patients was 51, three-fourths were women, and about half the patients were diagnosed with mild depression and the other half with moderately severe depression.

After four weeks of treatment, evaluations by the patients' doctors—and self-evaluations by the patients themselves—indicated that there was improvement or freedom from symptoms in about 80 percent of patients. As for the risks from St. John's wort, the data indicated that only 79 patients (2.4 percent of the total) experienced any side effects from the herb. Among the 48 patients (1.5 percent of the total) who dropped out of the study, 10 cited allergic reaction and four cited dizziness as the reason.

The most common side effect noted in this study, "gastrointestinal symptoms," was experienced by 0.55 percent of patients. (The study's authors note that about half these patients were experiencing gastrointestinal symptoms *before* the study began, suggesting that "a specific association with the treatment is somewhat questionable.") The second most common side effect was allergic reactions, mostly involving the skin, which affected 0.52 percent of patients. Those reactions, the authors suggest, may be related to the herb's photosensitizing properties (See the discussion of St. John's wort and photosensitivity reactions beginning on page 45.)

The authors contrasted the frequency of side effects in this study with results from previous studies in which standard antidepressants were assessed. They concluded that "the side effect rate is only about one-tenth, and the therapy dropout rate only about one-fifth, of those with synthetic antidepressants." This difference, they add, "should be a considerable contribution to good compliance during outpatient treatment."

Synthetic antidepressants work against depression, but in the process they often cause side effects that can signficantly impair a person's lifestyle. For anyone who wants relief from mild to moderate depression while avoiding the side effects so often associated with standard antidepressants, St. John's wort is definitely the preferred alternative.

❧ CHAPTER 5 ❧

How St. John's Wort Works Against Depression—and the Studies that Prove It

When clinical studies in the 1980's began to show that St. John's wort could relieve mild to moderate depression, it was inevitable that researchers would be intrigued: What is it about St. John's wort that enables it to do what it does so well—and to cause so few side effects in the process?

Uncovering the secrets of St. John's wort, however, has turned out to be an often frustrating scientific challenge. But as researchers continue to pursue *how* St. John's wort works, they've shown conclusively through clinical studies that it *does* work—and work well—in alleviating depression in patients. This chapter will tell you what's currently known about how St. John's wort works and summarize the studies that have so convincingly shown that it does.

FIFTY POSSIBLE SUSPECTS

When you take a synthetic drug like Prozac, you're swallowing several different chemicals along with it, including the gelatin that makes up the capsule and the fillers and binders that are used in the manufacturing process. But only one of those chemicals—fluoxetine—is an active ingredient, meaning it affects the functioning of the body. In the case of Prozac, this active ingredient increases levels of serotonin in the brain, which helps to alleviate depression.

Now contrast Prozac and its single active ingredient with St. John's wort, whose flowers and leaves contain as many as 50 different chemicals— at least a dozen of which are known to affect the body in one way or another. It's no wonder that researchers face a challenge in figuring out which one—or more likely, which *ones*—so successfully work against depression.

In 1984, Japanese researchers believed they had uncovered the answer. They reported that hypericin, the main ingredient in St. John's wort, inhibited monoamine oxidase—suggesting that hypericin was responsible for the antidepressant effect and that it worked the same way as Nardil and other monoamine oxidase inhibitor (MAOI) antidepressants. (See Chapter Four for more information on MAOIs.)

Until the past couple of years, the assertion that St. John's wort worked as an antidepressant by inhibiting monoamine oxidase was widely accepted. But recently that assumption has been questioned, since researchers who have tried to confirm hypericin's effect as an MAOI have been unable to do so. It now turns out that hypericin—long assumed to be the key ingredient in St. John's wort's usefulness in treating depression—*actually plays no role at all in St. John's wort's antidepressant effect.*

At first glance, this would seem to be alarming news. After all, the potency of nearly all St. John's wort products is expressed in terms of their hypericin content—in most cases, 0.3 percent hypericin by weight. But there's apparently no need to worry, since "hypericin-standardized" extracts still offer you the chemicals responsible for the herb's antidepressant effects. In numerous clinical trails, these St. John's wort extracts have proven their effectiveness in treating depression.

It turns out that *something* in St. John's wort may have some monoamine oxidase-inhibiting ability—but it has been attributed not to hypericin but to a group of chemicals known as flavonoids. The current thinking among researchers is that, if St. John's wort does have a monoamine oxidase-inhibiting effect, it must be very small. Most experts are now convinced that St. John's wort must be producing its antidepressant effect in one or more ways that don't include inhibiting monoamine oxidase.

Could St. John's wort work its magic against depression by doing what Prozac does—inhibit the reuptake of serotonin by neurons in the brain? Two recent laboratory studies found that St. John's wort could indeed prevent nerve cells from reabsorbing serotonin. But in both studies, the effect required a high dose of St. John's wort—higher, most likely, than would be possible to achieve in people taking the herb orally. Nevertheless, it remains possible that SSRI activity may in part account for St. John's wort's antidepressant ability.

Other studies suggest that St. John's wort can increase brain levels of dopamine—yet another important neurotransmitter and one whose brain levels are known to be increased by another class of antidepressants, the tricyclics. And recent work by researchers at the National Institute of Mental Health suggests that St. John's wort—even in very dilute amounts—could increase levels of an important neurotransmitter called gamma-amino-butyric acid or GABA. Low levels of GABA have been associated with both major depression and bipolar depression (manic depression).

Finally, some researchers have proposed a novel explanation for how St. John's wort relieves depression. They argue that St. John's wort might not directly affect the brain at all but instead may be exerting its antidepressant effect by acting on the immune system. This suspected link between depression and the immune system has emerged from work in the new field known as psychoneuroimmunology—the study of how the immune system, the nervous system, and the mind interact with each other.

These researchers suspect that the real "target" of St. John's wort may actually be certain blood cells, including the lymphocytes and monocytes, which play important roles in the body's immune response. These cells secrete potent chemical messengers known as cytokines, which are extensively involved in communication between cells both inside and outside the immune system—especially in the nervous system.

In preliminary studies on the blood of human volunteers, these researchers have found that St. John's wort strongly inhibits the ability of blood cells to secrete an important cytokine known as interleukin-6. This cytokine is suspected of causing depression in susceptible people—and St. John's wort may be providing relief by suppressing interleukin-6.

Although St. John's wort is now being studied intensively, the exact "mechanism" by which it relieves depression remains unknown. Researchers now believe that no single chemical action is responsible. Instead, they suspect that St. John's wort treats depression by affecting several different biochemical pathways, perhaps causing subtle changes in all of them. Although each such change by itself might not be sufficient to treat depression, the sum of their effects equals the antidepressant potency of Prozac and other drugs that act through a single biochemical pathway.

Indeed, such a multifaceted mode of action may help explain the remarkable freedom from side effects enjoyed by people taking St. John's wort. The herb's unequaled gentleness to the body may be due to the fact that it affects many biochemical pathways in subtle ways rather than profoundly altering one or two pathways, as is the case with most of today's synthetic antidepressants.

WHAT THE CLINICAL TRIALS SHOW

Although we still don't know *how* St. John's wort works in treating mild to moderate depression, there is no question that it *does* work. Over a period of nearly 20 years, St. John's wort has been tested on more than 3,000 patients enrolled in numerous European clinical studies. These studies have shown that St. John's wort is clearly superior to placebos and appears to be equal in effectiveness to synthetic antidepressants. In addition, virtually every study comparing the herb with a standard antidepressant has found that St. John's wort causes fewer side effects—and several studies have found that it causes fewer side effects than the placebos with which it has been compared!

St. John's wort has only recently received attention in the United States, in part because virtually all the clinical studies on the herb have been carried out in Europe, particularly Germany, and very few of them were published in English. Americans received their first real introduction to St. John's wort in 1994, when a prestigious U.S. medical journal, the *Journal of Geriatric Psychiatry and Neurology*, published a special supplement devoted entirely to St. John's wort. This supplement, "Hypericum: A Novel Antidepressant," contained 17 scientific research papers on the herb, including seven clinical studies assesssing its effectiveness as an antidepressant.

The editor of the journal—Michael A. Jenike, M.D., of Massachusetts General Hospital in Boston—wrote an accompanying editorial in which he acknowledged that "until three months ago, I had never heard of hypericum [the alternative name for St. John's wort]." But he then noted:

"In reviewing these papers and other literature, I have been impressed with the potential of this compound [St. John's wort] as a therapeutic agent in the treatment of mild to moderate depressive illnesses, the kind of depressions that predominate in outpatient medical practices . . ."

One of the studies to which Jenike referred—a randomized, double-blind, placebo-controlled clinical trial—gave results that are typical of the findings from 15 studies carried out over the past 20 years in which St. John's wort was compared with a placebo. This particular study, carried out by Austrian and German researchers, involved 105 male and female outpatients from three medical centers who had been diagnosed with mild depression. The patients were seen at the beginning of the study, before any treatment was given, and then after two and four weeks of treatment.

Patients were given either a placebo three times a day or three 300 mg tablets of a St. John's wort extract standardized to 0.3 percent hypericin. Improvement in depressive symptoms was evaluated by using a 17-item questionnaire, the Hamilton Depression Scale, which is filled out by the patients' doctors. In addition, the patients were questioned specifically about possible undesirable side effects from their treatment. A total of 89 patients (42 in the treatment group, 47 in the placebo group) completed the four-week study.

Two weeks after treatment began, improvement was noted in both the placebo group and the group treated with St. John's wort, although scores in the St. John's wort group were significantly better. By the end of four weeks, the differences between the two groups were even greater: There was only a modest amount of additional improvement among patients in the placebo group, while the group treated with St. John's wort had continued to improve steadily. Based on their scores on the Hamilton Depression Scale, 67 percent of the group (28 of 42 patients) treated with St. John's wort had responded positively after four weeks of treatment, compared with only 28 percent of the placebo group (13 of 47 patients).

In comparing the depression scale results for the placebo and St. John's wort groups following the four-week study, the researchers noted "a particularly impressive clinical improvement" in three areas: "depressive mood" (feelings of sadness, hopelessness, helplessness, worthlessness); "difficulty initiating sleep"; and "psychological anxiety." Separate questioning after four weeks of treatment revealed that sleep disorders, headaches, and fatigue occurred significantly less frequently among patients taking St. John's wort than among patients in the placebo group.

The researchers reported that "notable side effects were not found." And in fact, side effects of any kind affected more patients in the placebo group (three) than in the St. John's wort group (two).

The conclusion of the study: St. John's wort is "a low-risk antidepressant for treatment of mild and moderate depression, with the advantage of reliable antidepressant efficacy and a minimum of side effects."

ST. JOHN'S WORT VERSUS STANDARD ANTIDEPRESSANTS

Studies such as the one described above, in which St. John's wort was compared with a placebo, have clearly shown that the herb is effective in treating depression. But in addition, at least a half dozen clinical studies have compared St. John's wort with standard antidepressants.

In all of these studies, St. John's wort proved equal to the standard drug as an antidepressant and caused fewer side effects as well. We'll briefly review one such study, carried out in Germany and published in the 1994 supplement to the *Journal of Geriatric Psychiatry and Neurology*, which exemplifies the findings of studies in which St. John's wort has gone head-to-head against antidepressants with a well-established track record of effectiveness.

In this study, a St. John's wort extract was compared with imipramine, a tricyclic antidepressant. Imipramine's effectiveness has been demonstrated in more than 1,000 therapeutic trials over 35 years, and it is considered the classic "reference" drug—the one against which all new antidepressants are compared to get an idea of how effective they are. The St. John's wort product was an extract standardized to contain 0.3 percent hypericin; three 300 mg tablets were taken daily.

The study involved 130 patients and was "double-blind," meaning that neither the patients nor the researchers administering the drugs knew which drug the patients were taking. The patients were examined at the start of the study and were then evaluated after one, two, four, and six weeks of treatment at 20 different medical centers.

As with the trial described above in which St. John's wort was compared with a placebo, severity of depression in this study was measured using the Hamilton Depression Scale. But in addition, two other depression scales were used: the Clinical Global Impressions (CGI) scale and a self-assessment scale completed by the patients.

After six weeks of treatment, the values for the Hamilton Depression Scale fell similarly for patients in both the St. John's wort group and the imipramine group, indicating a roughly equal reduction in the severity of depression in both groups.

The CGI scale assesses three different depression factors: therapeutic effect, alteration in status at the end of treatment and change in severity of the illness. Similar improvements for all three factors occurred in both treatment groups—but for all three, improvement was slightly greater in the St. John's wort group. For example, 81.8 percent of patients were classified as having gotten better while taking St. John's wort versus 62.5 percent of patients who did so on imipramine; and no patients on St. John's wort experienced a worsening of their condition versus two patients who became worse while on imipramine.

The researchers also looked at results among subgroups of patients—those with mild, moderate, or more severe depression at the start of the study as indicated by their Hamilton scores. Among the 51 patients classified with severe depression, those taking St. John's wort did significantly better than those taking imipramine—in terms of improvement on both the Hamilton scale and on two parameters of the CGI scale (therapeutic effect and change in severity).

Regarding side effects, they occurred less often and were less severe in the group taking St. John's wort than in the imipramine group. Eight patients taking St. John's wort (or 11.9 percent of the group) experienced a total of 11 symptoms, the most frequent of which were dry mouth (four cases) and dizziness (two cases). A total of 22 symptoms were mentioned by 11 patients (16.2 percent of the group) who took imipramine; the most frequent were dry mouth (nine cases), followed by dizziness and anxiety (three cases each) and constipation (two cases). And while 10 of the 11 symptoms associated with St. John's wort were said to be mild, for imipramine the totals were 15 classified as mild, four as moderate, and three as severe side effects.

So far, studies comparing St. John's wort with synthetic antidepressants have matched it only with imipramine and other tricyclics and not with newer antidepressants such as Prozac. But since St. John's wort has proven equal to the tricyclics as an antidepressant—and since the tricyclics are at least as effective as Prozac—there's every reason to assume that St. John's wort works as well as Prozac.

A LANDMARK REVIEW

St. John's wort reached a pinnacle of respectability in 1996, when the prestigious *British Medical Journal* published a major study on the herb's effectiveness in treating depression. In this study, researchers pooled and then analyzed the results of 23 different randomized clinical studies that had been carried out on St. John's wort. These trials involved a total of 1,757 patients with mild to moderately severe depression.

Thirteen of the trials analyzed in the *British Medical Journal* article compared St. John's wort with a placebo—the standard way to assess a drug's effectiveness. Overall, 55.1 percent of patients receiving St. John's wort improved compared with only 22.3 percent of patients who improved while taking the placebo. The researchers concluded that St. John's wort was "significantly superior" to the placebo.

Equally important, St. John's wort held its own in studies comparing it with the standard antidepressants in treating depression. Five of the studies analyzed in the *British Medical Journal* study reported on the numbers of patients who were "treatment responders," meaning that the patients' depression improved during the course of the study. The authors of the study found that 63.9 percent of patients treated with St. John's wort were treatment responders compared with 58.5 percent of the patients who responded to the standard antidepressants. They also noted: "The scores on the Hamilton Depression Scale after treatment were slightly better in patients on single [St. John's wort] preparations than in those on standard antidepressants."

Not surprisingly, the authors concluded that St. John's wort "may work as well as other antidepressants." But they found that "the evidence is still insufficient because of the limited number of patients included in the trials." In all, only six clinical trials have compared St. John's wort with standard antidepressants; and these were small studies, with the largest involving a total of 135 patients.

To resolve the issue, the authors of the *British Medical Journal* study urged that additional trials be carried out to show conclusively whether St. John's wort is as effective as standard antidepressants. Now, thanks to the growing interest in St. John's wort, the National Institutes of Health will soon be sponsoring a major study that may resolve the issue once and for all.

This NIH-funded study of St. John's wort is a collaborative effort involving three NIH branches: the Office of Alternative Medicine, the National Institute of Mental Health and the Office of Dietary Supplements. The study's goal, according to an NIH announcement, is "to evaluate the efficacy and safety of hypericum as a potential treatment for depression, in order to determine its role in helping many Americans afflicted with depressive conditions."

The study, which is expected to begin in 1998 and last for three years, will be a multicenter trial, involving patients at five to 10 clinical sites around the country. It will enroll 336 patients who have been diagnosed with mild to moderate major depression. Those 336 patients will be assigned at random to one of three treatment groups, with 112 patients per group: a placebo group, a group taking a standard antidepressant (one of the SSRIs) and a group that will take St. John's wort. The study will be the first study in which St. John's wort has been compared with one of the SSRIs.

The initial phase of this two-phase study will last for eight weeks—considerably longer than the four- to six-week duration of most previous studies of St. John's wort. During these eight weeks, the patients will take three tablets daily of either the placebo, the SSRI, or St. John's wort. (Those on St. John's wort will take a tablet containing 300 mg of St. John's wort extract.) The study will be double-blind.

The patients will be evaluated before the study and after the eight weeks of treatment to see whether they improved and by how much. (The main tool for evaluating patients will be the Hamilton Depression Scale, referred to earlier; the lower the score, the better the patient's mental state.) These results will determine how the three compare in alleviating depression.

This eight-week first-phase of the trial is known as the "acute efficacy" phase, and it forms the crux of the NIH study. But it will also be followed by a second phase that will evaluate the longer-term effects of St. John's wort—something that no other study has yet done. For an additional four months, those patients who responded favorably to their treatment in the study's first phase will continue taking whatever they'd taken during the first phase—either the placebo, the SSRI, or St. John's wort. The purpose of this second phase is to gauge how well St. John's wort compares with the SSRI and the placebo as maintenance therapy for depression. (Patients treated with antidepressants are often "maintained" on the drug following recovery from their depressive episode, to preserve their improved mood or to prevent a recurrence of the depression.)

In describing its upcoming study of St. John's wort, the NIH spelled out its "research hypothesis"—what it expects its study to reveal about St. John's wort. The hypothesis itself makes for revealing reading, because it shows that the NIH is expecting big things from this humble herb:

"Acute efficacy [the study's first phase]: Patients treated with hypericum (900 mg per day) will achieve significantly lower final HAM-D-17 [Hamilton Rating Scale for Depression] scores at Week 8 than patients treated with placebo. Adverse effects will not differ significantly between the hypericum and placebo groups, and hypericum will be better tolerated than the SSRI.

"Long term [the study's second phase]: Patients treated with hypericum 900 mg per day will have fewer relapses than patients treated with placebo."

This first long-term study of St. John's wort should provide useful information on the herb's antidepressant ability. And it should help answer one of the remaining questions about St. John's wort: whether people taking the herb for extended periods of time experience any side effects that haven't turned up in the shorter (four to six weeks) studies that have been carried out up to now.

A NEW WAY TO TREAT DEPRESSION

The story so far is that St. John's wort is a safe and effective antidepressant, but researchers still don't understand how it works—which has prompted some experts to express concern. "We don't know why it works," Dr. Wayne Jonas, head of the National Institutes of Health's Office of Alternative Medicine, said recently. "This is a complex preparation with multiple chemical components to it, and we don't know what the mechanism of action is in its effect on depression."

What's interesting is that the same qualities—effective antidepressant, unknown mode of action—are looked on *favorably* when the medicine in question is a synthetic drug. In a 1995 article on antidepressants, the *Harvard Mental Health Letter* noted that "certain newer antidepressants, such as bupropion (Wellbutrin), have unknown mechanisms of action that may provide new biological insights into depression."

The fact is, psychopharmacology experts are excited by the possibility that St. John's wort will also offer new insights into depression—and they're hopeful that these insights could lead to treatment strategies undreamt of so far. One such expert is Jerry Cott, Ph.D., a Maryland-based psychopharmacologist who is involved in research on how St. John's wort affects brain chemistry.

Cott notes that our present understanding of depression's biochemical nature is based on what antidepressants are known to do in the brain: They all increase the levels of one or more of the brain's neurotransmitters, the chemicals that allow nerve cells to communicate with each other. The newer antidepressants increase neurotransmitter levels by preventing their reuptake by the neurons that have produced them. The success of these reuptake-inhibiting drugs—both in treating depression and generating profits—has prompted pharmaceutical companies to focus on developing even more antidepressants that work this way. But as a result, says Cott, little real progress has been made in improving the treatment of depression in the last 40 years, ever since the first tricyclics were marketed in 1957. "How many more of these potent and selective reuptake inhibitors do we really need?" asks Cott.

"In searching for the answer to how St. John's wort acts as an antidepressant," Cott says, "we may learn something new about depression itself." And that knowledge, he says, could lead to a new generation of antidepressants that are both milder and more effective than those available now.

While researchers search for the secret to St. John's wort's antidepressant action, millions of people are benefiting from the fact that it does work against depression and does so with notably few side effects. And as we'll see in the next chapter, its impressive therapeutic effects aren't confined to depression but extend to other problems including anxiety, insomnia, and seasonal affective disorder.

❧ CHAPTER 6 ❧

How St. John's Wort Works Against Anxiety, Insomnia, and Seasonal Affective Disorder

As you now know, St. John's wort has been generating headlines—and legions of new users—because it has proven remarkably effective against depression. But this focus on depression has tended to obscure some of the other important mental benefits that this medicinal herb offers.

For example, clinical studies of St. John's wort, plus user experience over many centuries, shows that it works in alleviating anxiety, an even more prevalent problem than depression. In addition, it has proven useful in treating insomnia—a problem affecting one of every three adults—as well as seasonal affective disorder. This chapter will tell you just what else St. John's wort can do above and beyond treating depression.

ANXIETY: MORE COMMON THAN DEPRESSION

Feeling anxious—butterflies in the stomach, heart in the throat—is something that all of us experience throughout our lives. Anxiety is an emotion that's hard to describe but all too tangible when we're experiencing it. It's a feeling akin to fear but without an actual, concrete threat to justify the fear.

Most of you can remember experiences that aroused acute anxiety—getting lost on that sixth-grade field trip to Washington, D.C., or arriving at the check-in line for your plane trip and realizing you have forgotten your ticket. But aside from the unpleasant experiences we associate with it, anxiety for most people is often a useful sensation that helps us cope with life. It makes sure we're prepared when we have to meet with the boss, makes us buckle down at final exam time, and gets us home in time for dinner. And it also helps us respond when we really are confronted with a genuine threat, such as a mugger on a dark street.

For millions of people, however, anxiety is a crippling rather than a constructive emotion. A person with an anxiety disorder may feel anxious most of the time, usually without any apparent reason. Or episodes of anxiety may occur only occasionally but be so intense that they terrify and immobilize him. Sometimes these feelings are so unbearable that people may cease participating in everyday activities if that helps them to avoid the anxiety.

As described more fully in Chapter One, in 1978 the German government assembled a group of experts, known as Commission E, to evaluate the safety and effectiveness of some 1,400 herbal drugs and to publish their findings in a series of monographs, or special reports. An herbal medicine approved by the commission can be prescribed and used like any other drug.

In its monograph on St. John's wort, published in 1984, the commission approved the herb not only for "depressive moods" but for "anxiety and/or nervous unrest." That news should be of interest to a lot of people, since anxiety disorders are the most common of all mental problems.

THE ANTI-ANXIETY DRUGS

Just as there are synthetic drugs for treating depression, such drugs are also available for treating anxiety. Until the 1950's, anxiety could only be treated with barbiturates, which had two potentially disastrous side effects: It was all too easy to overdose with them, and all too easy to become addicted.

Then, beginning in the mid-1950's, anxiety treatment was revolutionized through the introduction of much-improved compounds. First came meprobamate (Miltown and Equanil) and then the products that remain the standard treatments for anxiety: the benzodiazepines, a group of products that include Valium and Librium. Meprobamate and the benzodiazepines are collectively known as "minor tranquilizers," since they are less sedating, less addictive, and generally cause fewer side effects than the barbiturates. In recent years, the FDA has approved another type of minor tranquilizer, buspirone (BuSpar), which is even less sedating than other anti-anxiety drugs.

Because of their clear superiority to the barbiturates for treatment of anxiety, the benzodiazepines (immortalized as "Mother's Little Helper" by The Rolling Stones in a 1960's song) became extremely popular. But only after they became extensively used by anxiety-prone patients did it become clear that these minor tranquilizers caused problems of their own.

Valium, Librium, and the other benzodiazepines turned out to be capable of causing addiction, both psychological and physical. This risk is low if the drugs are used for short periods of time. But even with these precautions, some people turn out to be extremely sensitive to these drugs and become addicted to them even while on very low doses. Furthermore, the risk of addiction and other adverse effects from these drugs rises steeply when they're taken along with other drugs, especially alcohol.

Today, drugs for treating anxiety are usually reserved for people whose anxiety is triggered by a known cause and that is likely to last for just a short period of time. Examples of such situations include the death or illness of a family member or close friend or being laid off from a job. This means that, for the millions of people who suffer from more generalized anxiety, drugs for handling their condition really haven't been satisfactory—until now, with the widespread availability of St. John's wort.

ST. JOHN'S WORT TO THE RESCUE

When it comes to treating depression, the effectiveness of St. John's wort has been confirmed primarily by clinical studies in which the herb was compared either with a placebo or a standard antidepressant drug. As yet, however, similar studies have not been done to assess its effectiveness against anxiety. Instead, these anti-anxiety effects have been established through less direct, but still quite valid, ways. As it turns out, the clinical studies that established St. John's wort's usefulness against *depression* have also shed considerable light on its ability as an *anti-anxiety agent.*

When any herb or drug is tested in clinical studies on depression, researchers must be able to compare the mental state of patients before and after the study in order to determine whether this agent has been effective or not. The principal way of doing this is through use of the Hamilton Depression Scale. The scale consists of 17 items. For each item, researchers evaluating patients both before and after the study assign a score of one to five based on severity, with one indicating least severe illness.

The items consist mainly of the well-established symptoms of depression: guilt, suicidal thoughts, depressed mood, difficulty falling asleep, loss of sex drive—as well as anxiety. In fact, anxiety figures in two of the 17 questions.

One of those anxiety items is "psychic anxiety" (fearful thoughts, worry, tension, irritability, feeling jumpy) and the other is somatic anxiety, or anxiety expressed through physical changes including rapid pulse, gastrointestinal upset, or the need to urinate frequently. So St. John's wort's effectiveness against depression, as shown by its positive impact on the Hamilton Depression Scale, is partially a result of its ability to soothe anxiety. But there is also further evidence affirming St. John's wort's usefulness against anxiety.

When Germany's Commission E was asked to evaluate the usefulness of St. John's wort and other herbs, it was not restricted to looking at controlled clinical studies. Instead, the commission was asked to consider other types of data as well, including how the herb has been used historically, the clinical impressions of physicians regarding the herb's usefulness, and the opinions of patients who have tried the herb. The evidence in favor of St. John's wort as a treatment for anxiety was clear and convincing.

For centuries, folk healers have relied on it as a "nerve tonic," effective in treating numerous anxiety-related conditions including insomnia and agitation. And equally important, healers could recommend St. John's wort without hesitation because they knew there was little chance of unpleasant side effects from the herb.

The recent clinical studies on St. John's wort have confirmed what the herbal healers had discovered empirically over the course of centuries: that this herb has the power to calm people and to elevate their mood, and in general to dispel the anxiety-induced fogs that most all of us experience occasionally.

CAN YOU BENEFIT?

Anxiety is one of the most common symptoms of depression. If you're someone who suffers from mild or moderate depression in which anxiety is present, you and your doctor may well decide that St. John's wort is the ideal treatment. And St. John's wort may also be of help to you if you're one of the many people for whom anxiety rather than depression is the main emotional problem.

These sufferers include the millions of people who are mildly anxious but whose anxiety does not disrupt their daily life. This group would also include many other people whose anxiety is more severe. All these people have one of the "anxiety disorders," which include panic disorder, phobias such as social phobia and fear of heights, obsessive-compulsive disorder, and post-traumatic stress disorder. Knowledge already gained about

St. John's wort suggests that it might be particularly useful in treating one of these anxiety disorders, known as generalized anxiety disorder, or GAD.

People with GAD are *super* worry warts. They're afflicted with anxiety that is much more severe than the kind that all of us experience from time to time, and their worry and tension is both exaggerated and chronic. With psychotherapy, the underlying cause of such anxiety can sometimes be identified. But for most sufferers, the cause of their anxiety is unknown—and it makes their lives miserable, sometimes to the point where they have trouble functioning. Fortunately, most people with GAD are only mildly impaired by their anxiety and are usually able to function in most social situations and on the job.

GAD usually develops gradually. Most often it begins affecting people in childhood or adolescence, but sometimes it doesn't become noticeable until adulthood. It is more common in women than in men and often strikes relatives of people who are affected, suggesting an underlying genetic cause. People are diagnosed as having GAD if they have spent at least six months worrying excessively about a number of everyday problems. Fortunately, the symptoms of GAD usually diminish with age.

People with GAD are always expecting something disastrous to happen and often worry excessively about health, money, family, or work. They typically can't rid themselves of their concerns, despite the fact that they usually realize that they're overreacting to a particular situation. In addition, they're usually unable to relax and often have trouble both falling asleep and staying awake. Physical symptoms often accompany their mental anguish, and these include trembling, twitching, muscle tension, irritability, headache, sweating or light-headedness, or feeling out of breath.

Anti-anxiety medications such as Xanax and Valium can provide relief only for short-lived stressful periods and haven't been found to offer much help for the chronic anxiety of GAD. And if these medications are used for long periods, there is a real danger that the patient will become habituated to the drug and require larger and larger doses. Once the drug is stopped, the anxiety symptoms return in full force.

THE ST. JOHN'S WORT ADVANTAGE

Compared with anti-anxiety drugs, which are both ineffective and potentially dangerous treatments for GAD, St. John's wort seems to have some real advantages. Consider first of all the benefits it could offer GAD patients:

• *People with GAD seem unable to relax.* St. John's wort has a long history of making people feel more tranquil and at peace with themselves.

• *People with GAD have trouble falling asleep and staying asleep.* As we'll discuss later in this chapter, studies suggest that St. John's wort helps people achieve deeper, better-quality sleep.

• *People with GAD have trouble concentrating.* Studies indicate that St. John's wort improves the ability to concentrate as well as other cognitive abilities.

• *People with GAD sometimes also suffer from depression.* As this book makes clear, St. John's wort is notably effective in lifting mood and alleviating depression.

• *Most people with GAD are only mildly impaired by their anxiety.* St. John's wort's effectiveness against mild to moderate depression suggests that it might be especially appropriate for milder forms of anxiety disorder as well.

As far as safety is concerned, St. John's wort seems clearly superior to the anti-anxiety drugs. The studies to date have not found an instance of anyone having become habituated to St. John's wort. Furthermore, there are no published reports of anxiety returning in full force after treatment with the herb has stopped. St. John's wort seems particularly suited for treating GAD, since this is a chronic condition requiring a treatment that is safe enough to be taken for months or even years.

As yet, long-term clinical studies to assess St. John's wort's usefulness for treating GAD have not been done. But judging by the herb's long and distinguished record of safe use, it's unlikely that serious side effects from long-term use will turn up.

On the other hand, not enough is known about the herb's effectiveness against anxiety to recommend it for the often more severe types of anxiety disorders such as panic disorder or post-traumatic stress disorder. Such conditions can cause severe emotional distress and greatly restrict people's lives.

Many people with panic disorder, for example, are unable to leave their houses for fear of confronting a situation that will provoke anxiety. If you are one of these people, you should be under a doctor's care and should not rely on a treatment such as St. John's wort until more is known about its ability to quell severe anxiety problems. Or if you *do* plan to use the herb, first discuss it with your doctor to see if it's appropriate.

For the many people who are mildly anxious, St. John's wort may well be worth a try. Its effectiveness against anxiety has been established through centuries of use and, more recently, through clinical studies involving depressed patients for whom anxiety is often a symptom.

AN HERB FOR ALL SEASONS

Since St. John's wort is effective in treating mild to moderate depression, perhaps it's not surprising that it has shown promise in treating seasonal affective disorder (SAD), which can be thought of as an extreme form of the "winter blues." People with SAD are usually lethargic, sleep more than usual, have great difficulty getting up in the morning, and tend to overeat and have a craving for carbohydrates—which can result in significant weight gain over the winter months. SAD tends to run in families and affects an estimated 11 million Americans each year, 60 to 90 percent of them women.

Where you live plays a major role in susceptibility to SAD: the closer to the North or South Pole, the greater the incidence. People in the northern United States and Canada are eight times more likely to develop SAD than people living in sunny southern areas such as Florida.

Although it's not clear what causes SAD, the disorder may involve the neurotransmitter serotonin. Low serotonin levels are associated with depression, and serotonin levels fall to their lowest level in the brain during the short days of winter. Not surprisingly a common treatment for SAD is the use of Prozac and other selective serotonin reuptake inhibitors, which increase serotonin levels in the brain.

The standard treatment for SAD, however, is light therapy (also known as phototherapy), since SAD appears to be triggered by inadequate outdoor light reaching the eyes. In the most common form of phototherapy, people sit for 15 minutes to two hours a day in front of a light box that exposes them to a strong fluorescent light—up to a maximum of 10,000 lux, or 20 times brighter than ordinary indoor light. St. John's wort could be a useful addition—and perhaps an effective alternative—to light therapy.

In a study published in 1994, researchers investigated whether St. John's wort may also be useful for treating SAD, and whether taking the herb could help improve the effectiveness of light therapy. The four-week study involved 20 SAD patients (13 women and seven men). All of them were administered tablets containing St. John's wort extract (three 300 mg tablets daily). In addition, 10 of the patients received two hours of daily phototherapy with a bright white light (3,000 lux), while the other 10 received two hours of dim light (less than 300 lux) daily. (The 3,000-lux exposure corresponds to the amount of light received when looking out of a window on a spring day and is about five times brighter than normal room lighting.)

At the start of the study, both groups of SAD patients scored similarly on the Hamilton Depression Scale. Following the four weeks of treatment, the patients on St. John's wort and bright-light exposure had improved significantly, with their Hamilton score dropping by an average of 72 percent. Those patients on St. John's wort and dim-light exposure also improved significantly (a reduction of 60 percent on their Hamilton score).

In this study—the first ever to investigate the effectiveness of St. John's wort in SAD patients—the researchers concluded that St. John's wort exerts an antidepressive effect on patients with SAD. They also said that their results support the notion that the antidepressant effect of St. John's wort might be strengthened if SAD patients taking the herb were also treated with phototherapy.

THINK CLEARER THOUGHTS

Several studies have looked at the effect of St. John's wort on the functioning of the central nervous system. In these studies, subjects underwent electroencephalograms (EEGs, which measure electrical currents in the brain) before taking extracts of St. John's wort, and again after taking the herb daily for several weeks. In most of these studies, subjects similarly underwent tests of visual and auditory "evoked potentials." These studies indicate that St. John's wort acts in several ways to improve cognitive functioning.

In a 1994 study, healthy volunteers took St. John's wort daily for four weeks. Comparing the subjects' EEGs after four weeks of treatment with their appearance at the start of the study, the researchers found that the herb had caused enhanced activation in the theta and beta-2 regions of the EEG, which they interpreted as indicating that the herb produced a relaxing but not a sedative effect.

When the researchers looked at changes in evoked potential following treatment with St. John's wort, they found that the latency period—the time delay between administering the stimulus and the brain's response to it—had shortened considerably. This finding suggests that St. John's wort helps to quicken thinking ability, or what the researchers described as "more rapid general information processing by the brain."

IMPROVE YOUR SLEEP

Difficulty sleeping is perhaps the most common of all symptoms of depression. People who are depressed sleep fitfully and all too often awaken early. But in addition, insomnia affects an estimated one-third of nondepressed people as well, and is an especially common problem among the elderly. For centuries, St. John's wort has been recommended as a sleep aid, and more recent studies have provided scientific evidence for that effect.

In one of those studies, 12 older (average age 60), healthy female volunteers took three, 300 mg tablets of St. John's wort extract for four weeks and placebo tablets for another four weeks. The study was double-blind, so neither the researchers nor the patients knew which tablets were which. During the course of the study, each subject spent a total of four nights in a sleep laboratory, where recording devices measured rapid eye movement (REM) sleep and other stages of sleep.

The most notable result of administering St. John's wort to these older subjects was an increase in slow-wave sleep during two of the deep stages of sleep. Since people experience a decline in deep sleep as they get older, St. John's wort may be especially useful for improving sleep in older people.

In addition, this effect that St. John's wort has on deep sleep may contribute to its antidepressant effect, since a deficit in slow-wave sleep is an important indicator of depression and other mood disorders.

As yet, no clinical trials have been carried out on patients with insomnia comparing St. John's wort with a placebo or other drugs—the kind of study that is needed to show conclusively that a medicine is effective. But throughout history, folk healers have recommended this herb for its ability to improve sleep, while recent studies have added to the evidence. And based on my friend Carol's experience, St. John's wort is definitely something that a person with insomnia should seriously consider taking.

Carol, a 44-year-old businesswoman, has been suffering from insomnia as well as depression. When I told Carol that I would be writing a book on St. John's wort, she became interested in the herb and decided to try it. She promised me that she'd write down her impressions of the herb. This is what she had to say after taking a liquid extract of St. John's wort for six weeks:

> "My depression was triggered by a series of stressful events including a relationship ending and my mother's serious illness. I was suffering from a great deal of anxiety and had been living on two hours of sleep a night for many months. All this was on the heels of a divorce I hadn't yet recovered from and a three-year bout with irrita-

ble bowel syndrome. Plus my boss had just given me responsibility for supervising a special project.

"Basically, I was a mess. I was seeing my psychotherapist once a week but couldn't kick my feelings of hopelessness and loneliness. When I finally went to a psychiatrist for medication, I was near hysteria. He prescribed an antidepressant called Serzone, which I took for two years. For me, Serzone always seemed to help with my sleep and anxiety as much as it helped me as an antidepressant.

"I had been completely off Serzone for about four months when I started taking the St. John's wort. I wanted to try it because I was losing a lot of sleep again, getting only two or three hours for too many nights in a row. I wasn't depressed but was anxious about my work and feeling very lonely from working day and night all summer long on another big project. Above all, I was afraid of slipping into a deep depression again and wanted to try to prevent that.

"My experience with St. John's wort resembled what happened when I was taking Serzone. Almost immediately—within days—of taking St. John's wort, it started to help me sleep better, which really helped with my anxiety problems. Within a few weeks of starting on St. John's wort, I was consistently sleeping for longer periods of time every night. Now, after about six weeks of taking it, I'm sleeping like a baby. I sleep from six to eight hours every night, just like a real person— and this in spite of family problems and work in-

security and all the other things that normally keep me awake at night. That's how I know it's working: I would NEVER have been able to sleep with all that has been happening and not happening in my life over the past month.

"For example, the other night my sister-in-law picked up the extension while I was talking to my brother and screamed at me, called me names, and blamed me for her bad marriage. I was literally shaking when I got off the phone with her and thought that I'd never sleep that night. But I did! Even days later I was still disturbed at her behavior, but I slept well every night.

"I had read that St. John's wort takes longer to start working than synthetic antidepressants, but I don't think that was true in my case. It seemed to take effect as rapidly as the Serzone I'd been taking and may have even acted more quickly. In terms of side effects, there are absolutely none that I'm aware of from taking St. John's wort.

"I'm grateful for having found out about this gentle but effective herb. It has certainly changed my life for the better!

❧ CHAPTER 7 ❧

Your St. John's Wort Treatment Plan

If you've read the previous chapters, you know that St. John's wort may help to lift your depressed mood, soothe your anxiety, and help you sleep better. And you know that this medicinal herb is not only effective but is remarkably free of the side effects usually associated with synthetic antidepressant drugs.

Now that you know what St. John's wort can do for you—and what it won't do *to* you—it may be time for you to join the millions of other people who are already benefiting from this herb. This chapter will help you devise your own St. John's wort treatment plan. It tells you the kind of supplements to take, the doses that have been proven effective in clinical trials, and how long it may take for results to occur.

The chapter also explains why it's important to

buy only those products that have been "standard-ized" to contain a guaranteed amount of hypericin and tells you the recommended doses of St. John's wort that have proven to be both effective and safe in numerous clinical trials.

Finally, this chapter offers you the most comprehensive, up-to-date information available anywhere on St. John's wort products: a table listing brand names, where to obtain the products (in health food stores or by mail order), the names, addresses, and phone numbers of the companies selling them, the form in which they are sold (capsule, tablet, liquid, etc.), how the products are standardized, and their retail prices.

ADOPT OUR ANTIDEPRESSION STRATEGY

As effective as St. John's wort is in combating depression, it's just one part of our three-part antidepression strategy. You can greatly increase your chance for successful treatment if you not only take St. John's wort but adopt our recommendations regarding dietary and lifestyle changes.

As you'll see in Chapter Eight, what you eat or don't eat can have a major impact in determining whether you become depressed. Maintaining an adequate intake of the B vitamins, for example, is especially important for warding off depression and for alleviating depressed moods. This chapter tells you the foods that provide generous amounts of the B vitamins and also discusses other dietary components that can influence whether you become depressed, including antioxidants, carbohydrates, omega-3 fatty acids, alcohol, and caffeine.

Changing your lifestyle can also be crucially important both in warding off depression and handling depression successfully if it does occur. The changes you make don't have to be dramatic: Something as simple as starting on an exercise program can be be a tremendous help in reducing stress, one of the most important factors in triggering depression.

In Chapter Nine, we tell you about the types of exercise that are most useful against depression and tell you about relaxation exercises that can do wonders for your mental outlook. This chapter also discusses how certain medications and cigarette smoking can contribute to depression. And for anyone considering psychotherapy, the chapter discusses the qualifications of the different mental health professionals and describes the various therapies that benefit depressed people.

WORK WITH YOUR DOCTOR

If you're reading this book, there's a good chance that you're interested in St. John's wort because of its effectiveness in treating depression. As emphasized previously in this book, depression is a serious and potentially fatal illness. It should not be taken lightly—and neither should a decision to try St. John's wort.

If you are now taking an antidepressant drug and want to discontinue it in favor of St. John's wort, *be certain to consult with your doctor before doing so.* Withdrawing abruptly from a psychiatric drug can put you at risk for developing serious and even life-threatening emotional and physical reactions.

If your doctor agrees that it's all right for you to try St. John's wort, you'll probably have to be gradually weaned off the drug you're now taking as you begin taking St. John's wort. That can be a tricky business, putting you at risk for a possible relapse of your depression as well as headache, nausea, or other physical side effects. Don't try this balancing act by yourself; work in cooperation with your doctor.

And if you're already taking a synthetic antidepressant, don't try adding St. John's wort to your treatment regimen without consulting your doctor. As we explain in more detail in Chapter Three, St. John's wort could conceivably interact with standard antidepressants to cause high blood pressure and other problems.

Even if you're not currently taking an antidepressant drug but want to try St. John's wort, we recommend that you first consult with a healthcare professional. Since depression can be a serious illness, self-medicating yourself to treat it may pose a risk to your health.

Feeling that you need something to elevate your

mood may indicate that you're suffering from nothing more serious than a temporary case of the blues. But on the other hand, it could be an indicator that you're depressed—perhaps far more depressed than you realize.

The insidious thing about depression is that it can rob us of our ability to evaluate our own mental state objectively. The symptoms that you recognize as indicating that you're depressed could be just the tip of an unrecognized depression iceberg. So if you're thinking about taking St. John's wort, first have a consultation with your family doctor, a psychologist, or a psychiatrist.

If a routine check of your medical condition is called a physical, then the downturn in your mood may signal that you're due for a "mental." As emphasized repeatedly in this book, St. John's wort seems to be useful for mild to moderate depression, *but there is little evidence regarding its effectiveness against severe depression.* You may actually require a medication that is more potent than St. John's wort. If that's the case, then taking St. John's wort might actually keep you from receiving treatment that could end your depression or keep it from becoming worse.

BUY AN EXTRACT

Once you've decided to take St. John's wort, you next must decide which product to buy. Your local health food stores probably offer a large variety of St. John's wort products—the crude herb, liquid extracts, tablets, capsules, and teas. Our advice is to buy the herb in the form of an extract—which comes in both liquid and solid forms.

Extracts are the most potent form in which St. John's wort can be obtained. All of the clinical studies—some 25 in all—establishing St. John's wort's effectiveness in treating depression have used extracts, so it makes sense for you to use them too.

Extracts are the end result of an effort to "distill down" the plant into its medicinally useful ingredients. Ideally, an extract retains the same chemical profile as the original herb but in a much more concentrated form. An extract is not only much more potent than the original herb but also more palatable and easier to swallow.

BUY A *STANDARDIZED* EXTRACT

Buying an extract of St. John's wort that's not standardized is like buying a car and knowing nothing about its engine. You have no idea whether what you're buying has the potency to produce a therapeutic benefit. In the same way an eight-cylinder engine can assure you of adequate horsepower, standardization means the extract you're taking has a "guaranteed potency."

When an herbal extract is standardized, it means that the manufacturer has tested the extract to ensure that it contains a particular concentration of a key bioactive ingredient. Buying a standardized extract not only gives you an extract—the most potent form of St. John's wort—but also one with a known potency. (See the sidebar at the end of this chapter for a more detailed description of how extracts are made and standardized.)

In the case of St. John's wort, all solid and liquid extracts are standardized to contain a specified amount of hypericin, one of the herb's main ingredients. Hypericin was chosen because it was thought to be the ingredient responsible for the antidepressant effect of St. John's wort. As described in Chapter Five, researchers now know that hypericin plays no role in St. John's wort's antidepressant effect. Nevertheless, as clinical studies have proven, products standardized according to their hypericin content will also contain the key bioactive ingredients that *do* work to relieve depression. But if you buy one of the many nonstandardized St. John's wort products now being offered, you have no assurance that the proper ingredients are present—and in the amounts needed to be effective.

Most solid and liquid extracts of St. John's wort are standardized to contain 0.3 percent of hypericin by weight. So if you have a 300 mg capsule of St. John's wort extract that is standardized to 0.3 percent hypericin, that capsule will contain 0.3 percent times 300 mg, or 0.9 mg of hypericin.

Does an extract standardized to contain 0.3 percent hypericin also offer therapeutically useful levels of the other desirable St. John's wort ingredients? The evidence indicates that it does. In most of the recent clinical studies in which St. John's wort has been proven effective in treating depression, patients daily took capsules or tablets of St. John's wort extract that had been standardized to contain 0.3 percent hypericin. Many extract products that are standardized in this way are now available and are likely to work for you too. So we recommend that you buy a liquid or solid extract that has been standardized to contain a concentration of 0.3 percent hypericin.

Which particular standardized extract should you choose? That's difficult to say. In the clinical studies that have established St. John's wort's effectiveness in treating mild to moderate depression, one product—Jarsin 300—has been used more than any other, and it's now the best-selling antidepressant in Germany. Jarsin 300 is standardized to contain 0.3 percent hypericin and comes in tablets containing 300 mg of extract per tablet. Lichtwer Pharma, the German company that makes Jarsin 300, recently began marketing an identical product in the U.S. under the name Kira.

Since Kira has a history of effectiveness in clinical studies, Lichtwer Pharma justifiably labels it "the clinically proven hypericum formula (St. John's wort)." But Kira is also one of the most expensive St. John's wort products on the market: A box of 45 Kira tablets costs $15, or about a dollar a day for the recommended three tablets daily.

As you'll see in the table below, Kira now has many competitors that are essentially similar: extracts standardized to contain 0.3 percent hypericin and marketed in capsules or tablets containing 300 mg of extract. It's not possible at this time to recommend one brand over another, since head-to-head studies comparing different brands have not yet been done. But certainly the wisest course of action is to rely on brands of St. John's wort extract that, like Kira, are standardized to contain 0.3 percent hypericin. Most of the well-established dietary supplement makers—Solaray, Nature's Way, Standard Homeopathic, and others—now market St. John's wort in this formulation.

TAKE THE RIGHT DOSE . . .

No matter how miraculous the therapy, it won't make you feel better unless you take enough of it. As we've noted, clinical studies producing antidepressant benefits have used 300 mg solid-extract tablets standardized to contain 0.3 percent hypericin. Most of these studies used a daily dose of 900 mg of extract, meaning that patients took three 300 mg tablets daily. You may also want to start out on this dose, but should do so only in consultation with your doctor. (The National Institutes of Health has tacitly endorsed that dose as well: The U.S. multi-center trial of St. John's wort, sponsored by the NIH and set to begin in 1998, will also use 300 mg tablets of a St. John's wort extract standardized to contain 0.3 percent hypericin; and patients in this study will be taking three 300 mg tablets daily. This study is discussed in more detail in Chapter Five.)

But don't feel you have to limit yourself to a solid (capsule or tablet) form of St. John's wort extract. The standardized liquid extracts on the market should work as well as the tablets or capsules. (In a recent review of 25 controlled clinical studies involving St. John's wort extracts, seven of the studies used liquid extracts.) Several standardized liquid extracts of St. John's wort are listed in the table on page 138.

If you travel a lot or tend to be in a hurry most of the time, you may prefer the convenience of capsules or tablets over liquid extracts. A liquid extract will typically require that you measure out 75 drops per day (three 25-drop doses), which you'll want to dilute in water or some other liquid rather than take straight. That's not as simple or as quick as swallowing three tablets or capsules.

. . . BUT BE WILLING TO BE FLEXIBLE

Recommended doses are just that—recommendations—and they can be adjusted either upward or downward.

If for example, you don't feel an effect from an extract's recommended dose of three 300 mg tablets per day, it's probably safe to try taking a higher dose—especially in light of this herb's impressive history of safe use. One factor to consider is your body weight: The bigger you are, the higher the dose you may require.

Our advice is to take the recommended dose of St. John's wort for four weeks. For capsules and tablets containing St. John's wort extract, that will generally be three capsules or tablets per day. If you have started to notice some improvement in your mood by that time, try cutting back to two doses per day rather than three. You want the lowest daily dose that will be effective so as to minimize the risk of side effects. Older people in particular may find that they can reduce their dosage of St. John's wort and still experience the herb's benefits.

On the other hand, you should consider going above the starting dose if you haven't noticed any improvement after taking the recommended dose for four weeks. Since extracts are the most potent form of St. John's wort, you should be careful not to greatly exceed the recommended dose. But it's probably safe, for example, to go from the recommended dose of three tablets per day to four per day.

BE ALERT FOR SIDE EFFECTS

No matter what dose you're taking, cut back on St. John's wort if you think it might be causing complications. If side effects are severe, stop taking the herb immediately and consult your doctor. Fortunately, most side effects associated with St. John's wort are mild and tend to diminish as your body becomes accustomed to the herb.

Sometimes all it takes to handle a mild side effect (upset stomach, for example) is to cut back slightly on your daily dose. Alternatively, try taking the herb with meals and with a large glass of water as a chaser.

BE PATIENT

Once you start taking St. John's wort, don't expect immediate results. It generally takes the synthetic antidepressants from two to six weeks to start producing results, and it's unrealistic to expect that St. John's wort will work any faster. Some people do begin to feel some effect on their mood within two weeks of starting on St. John's wort, but you shouldn't be surprised if it takes longer.

It's a good idea to take the herb for at least six weeks before giving up on it. Of course, that doesn't mean you *must* stick with St. John's wort during that time. As stated, St. John's wort is especially suitable for treating mild to moderate depression, and you may need a more potent treatment, such as one of the synthetic antidepressants, to handle your problem.

WHEN TO STOP

"How long should I take St. John's wort?" may well be the most frequently asked question about this herb and also the most difficult to answer. Fortunately, episodes of depression don't last forever. They typically abate after about three months, whether or not a person is treated for the problem. If St. John's wort has successfully improved your mood, you can certainly consider stopping it; but if you do, it's probably best to taper off gradually.

Whether it's safe to use St. John's wort for long stretches—several months or even years at a time, for example—is unclear, since clinical studies involving St. John's wort have generally lasted for just four to six weeks. The NIH-sponsored clinical trial of St. John's wort, mentioned above, should shed some light on whether longer-term use of the herb poses any risks. (See the Q and A's in Chapter Eleven for more information about how long you should consider using St. John's wort.)

OTHER FORMS OF ST. JOHN'S WORT

St. John's wort products come in many different forms. The extracts are definitely the best bet for anyone wishing to obtain help for depression, anxiety, or other mood disorders. Nevertheless, other forms of St. John's wort—the crude herb as well as teas, tinctures, and oils—serve useful purposes as well.

The remainder of this chapter will tell you about these other forms of St. John's wort, what they're most suited for, and—in the case of the tinctures, teas, and oils—how to make them yourself. We'll even tell you how to go about cultivating your own St. John's wort from seeds.

The crude herb consists of the flowers, buds, and upper leaves of St. John's wort that have been been dried and then chopped up or powdered. It can be bought in bulk quantities and is also available in capsules and tablets. The crude herb is usually relatively inexpensive; but its medicinal value is questionable for several reasons.

The chemical composition of crude herbs can vary greatly depending on when the herb was harvested, the weather, which parts of the herb were used, and other factors. And even under optimal conditions, the bioactive chemicals in crude St. John's Wart are present in such dilute amounts that you'd have to consume impractically huge amounts of the herb to gain any therapeutic benefit. Finally, when herbs are dried and sold in powdered or chopped-up form, their chemical constituents tend to degrade quickly, reducing the product's therapeutic potential even more.

Recommendation: Taking St. John's wort orally as a crude herb probably won't do much for you at all. The crude herb is best reserved for making your own tea, tincture, or oil.

Teas. Before high-potency tablets and capsules of St. John's wort were introduced several years ago, the millions of Europeans using St. John's wort relied mainly on a tea prepared from the leaves and flowering tops of the herb. The tea is prepared by pouring one cup of boiling water over one to two heaping teaspoonfuls (two to four grams) of the crude herb and allowing it to steep for about 10 minutes. More conveniently, you can also buy St. John's wort in tea bags. The recommended consumption is one to two cups per day over an extended period of time—four weeks at least.

Recommendation: Teas are certainly better than swallowing the crude herb when it comes to obtaining the medicinal ingredients in St. John's wort. But water may not be the best solvent for "pulling" those ingredients out of the plant so that they're available to be swallowed. In short, don't rely on St. John's wort tea to provide much therapeutic benefit against depression or other mood disorders.

Tinctures. St. John's wort tinctures are probably somewhat more potent than the teas because their solvent—an alcohol and water mixture—is assumed to absorb more of the herbal ingredients than water alone. Tinctures are made by soaking the crude herb in the solvent.

If you want to make your own St. John's wort tincture, start with the crude herb (see table following for the name of a company that supplies the raw herb) and a clean jar with a tight-fitting lid.

You'll also need a solvent (technically known as the menstruum) to produce your tincture. If you're using dried St. John's wort, choose 80 to 100 proof alcohol such as brandy, vodka or gin. With the fresh herb, use 190 proof grain alcohol. *Never use rubbing (isopropyl) alcohol!*

Chop the herbs finely by hand or put them into a food blender, and then transfer the chopped-up herbs to the clean jar. The herb material should occupy about one-half the volume of the jar (three-fourths if you are using fresh herbs). Then pour the alcohol over the herbs so that it completely covers them.

In the case of dried herbs, you'll need to add more alcohol over the next day or two, since the dried herbs will absorb much of the alcohol. Make sure that the plant material is covered with at least two inches of liquid. But if you're using fresh St. John's wort, your next addition should be water rather than alcohol—again, enough to keep the herbs covered with at least two inches of liquid. (If you don't add water, your fresh-herb tincture will have a very high alcohol content.)

Then, with the jar's cover screwed on tightly, shake the jar well. Place the jar in a dark place and allow the St. John's wort to soak (macerate, in herbal lingo) for four to six weeks—making sure that you shake the jar daily during that time.

After the four to six weeks of soaking, it's time to strain the contents of the jar. Use a large screen and line it with fine mesh cloth. After filtering the jar's contents, wring out the cloth so you get every last drop. Then bottle your tincture in dark bottles, in order to minimize damage from the sun. Stored in a cool dark place, your St. John's wort tincture should last for years.

Recommendation: Most tinctures are 1:5 herbal concentrates, meaning that they consist of one part herb (in milligrams) for every five parts of solvent (in milliliters). Expressed another way, about 80 percent of a tincture consists of alcohol and water and only about 20 percent is herbal material. That makes tinctures somewhat more potent than teas, but relatively dilute nonetheless.

Tinctures of St. John's wort are more potent than teas and should be able to provide some help in lifting a depressed mood. But unless you have access to sophisticated analytical equipment, you won't be able to standardize your home-made tinctures—so you can't be sure how concentrated your tincture is, nor what dose will be optimal. (The standard dose for St. John's wort tinctures is 20 to 30 drops taken four times a day.) If you prefer your St. John's wort in liquid form, you're probably better off using one of the standardized liquid extracts rather than a tincture.

Oils. St. John's wort oil has long been relied on for numerous external uses. The oil helps to soothe and heal hemorrhoids, superficial wounds, and other skin problems. Germany's Commission E, for example, has approved external St. John's wort preparations for use in treating skin abrasions, muscular pain, and first-degree burns. It is also reportedly quite useful in minimizing the irritation and burning that can result from radiation treatment. And when rubbed on the skin, St. John's wort works as a good massage oil and helps to ease the pain of sports injuries.

You can buy St. John's wort oil in stores or by mail order, and several of them are listed in the table on page 138. Or you can make your own oil. In fact, one of the best uses for St. John's wort that you have grown or harvested yourself is to make St. John's wort oil from it.

Typically, only the flowers of St. John's wort are used in making oils, and the oil most commonly used is olive oil. The standard way to make St. John's wort oil—soaking the flowers in oil and "infusing" the mixture in the sun—dates at least to the publication of the first edition of Gerard's *Herbal* in 1597.

To make your own St. John's wort oil, cut up or mash one cup of the fresh flowering tops, and place them in a lidded jar; then cover them with olive oil and put on the lid. Place the container in the sun and shake the jar once a day for two to three weeks. By now the oil should have developed its characteristic beautiful deep-red color. Press and strain the plant material from the oil, and store the oil in a dark, closed container in a cool area.

Alternatively, some experts recommend a shortcut method for making St. John's wort oil in which the flowers are soaked in the oil at a temperature of 45° C (113° F) for 10 days. Perhaps the fastest way to make St. John's wort oil is to heat the mix-

ture of flowering tops and olive oil at 70° C (158°
F) for 12 to 24 hours.

GROW AND HARVEST YOUR OWN?

St. John's wort can readily be grown from seeds.
It's an herbaceous perennial, meaning it should
bloom year after year, and it's also very hardy—
famous, in fact, for being able to thrive even in
inhospitable soil. (As mentioned earlier, St. John's
wort is considered a weed in some parts of the
world.) Sandy soil provides a good base for sowing
the seed. After sowing, be sure to water the seeds
occasionally. When seedlings appear, transplant
or thin them so that the plants are about two feet
apart.

The herb flowers in the summer, with petals
that are yellow to yellowish-brown in color. Harvesting for medicinal purposes is best done in July
or August. The parts to harvest are the flowering
tops of the plant, including the the middle to top
leaves, the unopened buds, and the flowers. These
parts of the plant contain the highest concentrations of hypericin, flavonoids, and other chemicals that are believed chiefly responsible for the
herb's beneficial effects. Optimally, these flowering tops should be gathered immediately before
the buds open or just after, so that you'll have a
mixture of buds and blossoms.

St. John's wort seeds can be ordered as "Hypericum perforatum seeds" by mail order from

Sheffield's Seed Catalogue in Locke, NY (315-497-1058). The minimal purchase is one pound of the seeds for $69.50.

Whether you grow your own St. John's wort or rely on plants that grow wild, take some precautions when harvesting it. There are reports of people developing skin sensitivity reactions, including blisters on the eyelids and forehead, from collecting St. John's wort. So it's a good idea to keep your hands covered while collecting the herb and to avoid contact with eyes and unprotected skin. If you want to use the fresh herb—to make a tincture out of it, for example—you should process it as soon as possible after harvesting.

As for the best way to dry St. John's wort, researchers in the past few years have compared several different methods to find which one was most successful in preserving the most important ingredients. They concluded that the best procedure for preserving the herb's constituents is to dry the herb in an oven at 70° C (158° F.) for 10 hours.

Once the herb is dried, it's very important to protect it from light so that the herb's active ingredients are not degraded. It can then be used in several ways—in teas, tinctures, or oil for external use.

HOW EXTRACTS ARE MADE AND STANDARDIZED

The process of making a solid or liquid extract of St. John's wort begins with the harvesting of its flowering tops—the flowers, the unopened buds, and the upper leaves of the herb. The chopped-up (and usually dried) crude herb is then combined with a solvent such as alcohol.

The crude herb is soaked in the solvent for a specified period of time—from several hours to several days, depending on the herb. During that time the solvent pulls, or extracts, the herb's key ingredients—its bioactive chemicals—from the dried plant and into the liquid. The solid residue is then filtered out, and you are then left with a dilute herbal liquid known as a tincture.

Liquid extracts are made by taking tincture material and processing it further, evaporating off some of the alcohol and leaving an alcohol-based liquid extract. (When a liquid extract with a nonalcoholic base is desired, a manufacturer will distill off all the alcohol and replace it with another liquid, most often glycerin.)

A solid extract of St. John's wort is made by taking the liquid extract and evaporating off all of the solvent, so that what is left is a dry, solid extract that contains a high concentration of the herb's active ingredients. If it's not already powdery, this substance may then be ground up until it's in the form of a fine powder. The solid extract is then packaged into the capsules and tablets marketed as St. John's wort extract. This is the main way that St. John's wort is sold—and makes St. John's wort products much more uniform in quality when compared with most other herbs you can buy.

Most of these other herbs are also sold as liquid or solid extracts. But even though you're buying them in a concentrated form, you don't really know whether the active ingredients in one bottle of Brand A's capsules, for example, are present at the same levels as in another bottle of the same brand. That's because different batches of virtually identical plant material can differ greatly in chemical composition—a "quality control" problem due to genetic differences among plants of the same species, soil fertility, temperature, length of the growing season, when the herb was harvested, and other factors. Even slight variations in processing the herb can produce major differences in the final product. Some key chemicals in herbs are extremely sensitive to heat, for example, and may be destroyed unless the temperature at which the herb is processed is strictly regulated.

Compared with the "purity" of synthesized drugs, this lack of quality control—this inability to know whether key chemicals are present in amounts adequate to exert a medicinal effect—has prevented herbal products from being accepted as legitimate treatments. But fortunately, over the past few years, manufacturers of St. John's wort and a few other important medicinal herbs have largely compensated for this problem. They've succeeded in producing herbal products of uniform potency through a process known as standardization.

Standardization involves analyzing several batches of extract to determine the concentration in each of a key bioactive ingredient. Then, by a process of adjustment—which usually involves mixing together various amounts of different batches—the manufacturer produces an extract that contains the desired concentration of this key ingredient.

Standardization yields tablets, capsules and liquids with a uniform potency, which allows more accurate doses to be given. In the case of St. John's wort, all standardized solid and liquid extracts are adjusted to contain a specified amount of hypericin—typically, 0.3 percent hypericin.

The table below offers a comprehensive list of five categories of St. John's wort products—tablets and capsules, liquids, teas, oils, and the crude herb. For each product, the table also lists the manufacturer, the retail price, and where the product can be obtained—health food store, drug store, retail chain store or by mail order.

The material in this table is based on information obtained from product catalogs, product labels, and interviews with manufacturers. No testing has been done to verify whether the claims made for these products—that they're standardized or contain a certain amount of extract, for example—are accurate. Finally, the information in this table should not be construed as an endorsement for any particular brand or brands of St. John's wort.

Table 2
St. John's Wort Products

TABLETS AND CAPSULES
Product Name: St. John's Wort Positive Mood Enhancer
Manufacturer: Amerifit; Bloomfield, CT; 800-242-3476
Form: Tablet
Standardization: 0.3% hypericin
Amount per capsule/tablet (mg): 300 mg
Capsules/tablets recommended daily: one tablet three times daily
No. of capsules/tablets per bottle: 60
Retail price: $9.99
Comments: Sold in drug stores nationwide.

Product Name: St. John's-Power
Manufacturer: Nature's Herbs; American Fork, UT; 801-363-4060
Form: Capsule
Standardization: 0.14% hypericin
Amount per capsule/tablet (mg): 250 mg
Recommended daily dose: one capsule two times daily
Amount of liquid per bottle: 60

Retail price: $9.99

Comments: Also available: St. John's-Power
    0.3% (standardized to 0.3% hypericin, 250
    mg per capsule, bottle of 90 capsules for
    $13.49). Both products sold in health food
    stores and by mail order from retailers,
    including L&H Vitamins, New York, NY
    (800-221-1152), Harvest Moon Natural
    Foods, Olathe, KS (800-466-3458), and
    Wealth of Health, Idaho Falls, ID (800-605-
    5235).

Product Name: St. John's Wort Complete

Manufacturer: Futurebiotics; Hauppauge, NY;
    516-273-6300

Form: Capsule

Standardization: 0.3% hypericin

Amount per capsule/tablet (mg): 125 mg

Recommended daily dose: two capsules "as
    needed"

Amount of liquid per bottle: 60

Retail price: $10.19

Comments: Also contains vitamins and amino
    acids.

Product Name: St. John's Wort

Manufacturer: Solaray; Park City, UT; 800-447-
    6527

Form: Capsule

Standardization: 0.3% hypericin

Amount per capsule/tablet (mg): 300 mg

Recommended daily dose: one to three
    capsules daily

Amount of liquid per bottle: 120
Retail price: $14.99
Comments: Available in health food stores.

Product Name: St. John's Wort
Manufacturer: Nature's Way; Springville, UT;
     801-489-1520
Form: Capsule
Standardization: 0.3% hypericin
Amount per capsule/tablet (mg): 300 mg
Recommended daily dose: one to two capsules
     daily
Amount of liquid per bottle: 90
Retail price: $11.99
Comments: Available in health food stores.

Product Name: St. John's Wort Herb
Manufacturer: Solgar Vitamin and Herb Co.;
     Leonia, NJ; 201-944-2311
Form: Capsule
Standardization: 0.3% hypericin
Amount per capsule/tablet (mg): 175 mg
Recommended daily dose: one to three
     capsules daily
Amount of liquid per bottle: 60
Retail price: $9.20
Comments: Each capsule also contains 300 mg
     of raw St. John's wort herb powder.
     Available only in health food stores.

Product Name: St. John's Solution Plus
Manufacturer: Quantum; Eugene, OR; 800-448-
     1448

Form: Tablet
Standardization: 0.3% hypericin
Amount per capsule/tablet (mg): 300 mg
Recommended daily dose: one to three per day
Amount of liquid per bottle: 60
Retail price: $13.99
Comments: Also sold in gelcap form (bottle of 48 for $14.99). Both products sold in health food stores, chain drug stores, chain retail stores, and by mail order.

Product Name: St. John's Wort
Manufacturer: Herbal Harvest, Inc.; Bohemia, NY; 516-567-9500
Form: Capsule
Standardization: 0.15% hypericin
Amount per capsule/tablet (mg): 300 mg
Recommended daily dose: one capsule three times daily
Amount of liquid per bottle: 100
Retail price: $11.99
Comments: Sold in pharmacies.

Product Name: St. John's Wort
Manufacturer: Elixir Tonics & Teas; Los Angeles, CA; 1-888-4TONICS
Form: Capsule
Standardization: 0.3% hypericin
Amount per capsule/tablet (mg): 300 mg
Recommended daily dose: three capsules per day
Amount of liquid per bottle: 90

Retail price: $17.00
Comments: Available by mail order from the
    company and in some retail outlets,
    including Nordstrom's.

Product Name: St. John's Wort
Manufacturer: Schiff; Salt Lake City, UT; 800-
    526-6251
Form: Capsule
Standardization: 0.3% hypericin
Amount per capsule/tablet (mg): 600 mg
Recommended daily dose: one capsule per day
Amount of liquid per bottle: 60
Retail price: $20
Comments: Available by mail order and in
    health food stores nationwide.

Product Name: St. John's Wort
Manufacturer: Nature's Bounty; Bohemia, NY;
    516-244-2000
Form: Capsule
Standardization: 0.15% hypericin
Amount per capsule/tablet (mg): 300 mg
Recommended daily dose: one to three
    capsules per day
Amount of liquid per bottle: 100
Retail price: $14.95
Comments: Sold in Walgreen's and other chain
    drug stores and by mail order from the
    company's Puritan's Pride mail-order
    division (800-645-1030). A higher-strength

product (0.3% hypericin, 100 capsules for $20.95) is also available by mail-order.

Product Name: Hyland's Hypericum
Manufacturer: Standard Homeopathic; Los Angeles, CA; 800-234-8879
Form: Tablet
Standardization: 0.3% hypericin
Amount per capsule/tablet (mg): 300 mg
Recommended daily dose: two tablets three times a day
Amount of liquid per bottle: 60
Retail price: $12.95
Comments: Sold in most health food stores and by mail order from the company

Product Name: Kira
Manufacturer: Lichtwer Pharma U.S., Inc.; Pittsburgh, PA; 412-928-9334
Form: Tablet
Standardization: 0.3% hypericin
Amount per capsule/tablet (mg): 300 mg
Recommended daily dose: one tablet three times a day
Amount of liquid per bottle: 45
Retail price: $15.00
Comments: Sold in Walmart, Kmart and other chain stores. This is the U.S. version of Lichtwer Pharma's Jarsin 300 (also known as LI 160), the brand used in most of the European clinical studies that have been carried out on St. John's wort.

Product Name: HyperiCalm
Manufacturer: Enzymatic Therapy; Green Bay, WI; 800-783-2286
Form: Capsule
Standardization: 0.3% hypericin
Amount per capsule/tablet (mg): 300 mg
Recommended daily dose: one capsule three times daily
Amount of liquid per bottle: 60
Retail price: $13.50
Comments: Available in health food stores nationwide. Enzymatic Therapy markets the same product under the name St. John's Wort Extract.

Product Name: St. John's Wort
Manufacturer: Natrol; Chatsworth, CA; 800-326-1520
Form: Capsule
Standardization: 0.3% hypericin
Amount per capsule/tablet (mg): 100 mg
Recommended daily dose: two capsules daily
Amount of liquid per bottle: 60
Retail price: $9
Comments: Contains several other herbs as well. Available in drug stores/health food stores nationwide. Call company for the name of the nearest store in your area that carries Natrol products.

Product Name: Hypericum Verbatim
Manufacturer: Hypericum Buyer's Club; Los
  Angeles, CA; 888-497-3742
Form: Tablet
Standardization: 0.3% hypericin
Amount per capsule/tablet (mg): 300 mg
Recommended daily dose: three tablets per day
  with meals
Amount of liquid per bottle: 280
Retail price: $27.50
Comments: Hypericum is the scientific name for
  St. John's wort. Tablets are scored so dose
  can be adjusted. Available by mail order
  from the company and in some health food
  stores.

Product Name: St. John's Wort
Manufacturer: Nature's Sunshine; 800-223-8225
Form: Capsule
Standardization: 0.3% hypericin
Amount per capsule/tablet (mg): 300 mg
Recommended daily dose: three capsules per
  day
Amount of liquid per bottle: 100
Retail price: $26.40
Comments: A multilevel marketing product
  available only through Nature's Sunshine
  distributors and managers. Call the toll-free
  number for the name of a representative
  near you.

Product Name: St. John's Wort
Manufacturer: Source Naturals; Scotts Valley,
  CA; 800-815-2333
Form: Tablet
Standardization: 0.3% hypericin
Amount per capsule/tablet (mg): 300 mg
Recommended daily dose: three tablets per day
Amount of liquid per bottle: 60, 120, 240
Retail price: $8.79, $16.39, $31.49
Comments: Product also available in capsules
  costing slightly more ($9.59, $17.89, $33.49).
  Available in health food stores nationwide,
  from health care professionals, and by mail
  order from several vitamin retailers
  including The Vitamin Shoppe (New Jersey),
  800-223-1216; Swanson's Health Products
  (North Dakota), 800-437-4148; Health and
  Vitamin Express (California), 800-848-2808.

Product Name: St. John's Wort Extra Strength
Manufacturer: Yerba Prima; Ashland, OR; 800-
  488-4339
Form: Capsule
Standardization: 0.3% hypericin
Amount per capsule/tablet (mg): 300 mg
Recommended daily dose: one tablet twice
  daily
Amount of liquid per bottle: 60, 180
Retail price: $9.95, $24.95
Comments: Yerba Prima also markets a lower-
  strength capsule, St. John's Wort Extract,

standardized to 0.14% hypericin and with 250 mg of extract per capsule; bottles of 60 and 180 capsules cost $7.95 and $19.95, respectively. Products are available in most health food stores and by mail order from the company. Rather than call, company prefers that you contact them in writing (740 Jefferson Ave., Ashland, OR 97520-3743) or by e-mail (yerba@yerba.com.)

LIQUIDS
Product Name: St. John's Wort Flower Buds
Manufacturer: Gaia Herbs, Inc.; Harvard, MA; 800-831-7780
Form: liquid extract
Standardization: one mg of hypericin/ml (equal to 0.9 mg of hypericin per usage)
Recommended daily dose: 25 drops three times daily between meals
Amount of liquid per bottle: 1 oz. (30 ml) per bottle (15-day supply)
Retail price: $29.95
Comments: This concentrated "guaranteed bioextractive" formula is made from the fresh herb. Available in health food stores and by mail order from the company.

Product Name: St. John's Wort Flowerbuds
Manufacturer: Gaïa Herbs, Inc.; Harvard, MA; 800-831-7780
Form: liquid extract
Standardization: not standardized
Recommended daily dose: 25 drops three times daily

Amount of liquid per bottle: 1 oz., 2 oz. 4 oz., 8 oz.

Retail price: $9.95, $18.95, $35.80, $67.75

Comments: Extract is made from the fresh herb. Available in health food stores and by mail order from the company.

Product Name: Fresh St. John's Wort Flowerbuds

Manufacturer: Gaia Herbs, Inc; Harvard, MA; 800-831-7780

Form: liquid extract

Standardization: 0.5 mg/ml of hypericin

Recommended daily dose: 25 drops three times daily

Amount of liquid per bottle: 1 oz.

Retail price: $15.95

Comments: This "standardized full-spectrum" extract is made from the fresh herb. Available in health food stores and by mail order from the company.

Product Name: St. John's Wort

Manufacturer: Nature's Answer; Hauppauge, NY; 516-231-5522

Form: liquid

Standardization: a minimum of 0.2 mg hypericin per milliliter

Recommended daily dose: 25-30 drops (1 ml.) three times daily

Amount of liquid per bottle: 1 oz.

Retail price: $8.99

Comments: Sold in health food stores. Liquid base contains 55-60% alcohol and coconut glycerin; also available in a non-alcohol formulation costing $9.99.

Product Name: St. John's Wort
Manufacturer: Herb Pharm; Williams, OR; 800-348-4372
Form: liquid extract
Standardization: Not standardized
Recommended daily dose: 2 to 5 times a day take 30-40 drops in a little water
Amount of liquid per bottle: 1 oz., 4 oz., 8 oz. 16 oz., 32 oz.
Retail price: $9.50, $36.10, $68.40, $129.20, $243.20
Comments: Although not standardized, this extract has been found to contain approximately 0.1% hypericin. Available by mail order from the company and in health food stores.

Product Name: St. John's Wort Herb
Manufacturer: Mountain Rose Herbs; North San Juan, CA; 800-879-3337
Form: liquid extract
Recommended daily dose: 10-60 drops one to four times daily.
Amount of liquid per bottle: 1 oz., 4 oz.
Retail price: $7.75, $24.50
Comments: Non-standardized extract made at a 1:1 concentration. Available only by mail order.

Product Name: St. John's Wort-Hypericum
Manufacturer: Wise Woman Herbals, Inc.;
    Creswell, OR; 800-532-5219
Form: liquid extract
Recommended daily dose: 10-60 drops one to
    four times daily
Amount of liquid per bottle: 1 oz., 2 oz., 4 oz.,
    8 oz., 16 oz.
Retail price: $9.00, $16.60, $30.60, $57.60,
    $108.00
Comments: Non-standardized extract made at a
    1:1 concentration. Available in some stores
    but primarily by mail order.

Product Name: St. John's Wort Herbal Actives
Manufacturer: Nature's Plus; Melville, NY; 800-
    645-9500
Form: liquid
Standardization: 0.3-0.5% hypericin
Recommended daily dose: 1 ml (1 dropperful
    or 20 drops) daily
Amount of liquid per bottle: 30 ml per bottle
    (30 day supply)
Retail price: $7.99
Comments: Sold in drug stores and health food
    stores.

TEAS
Product Name: Caffeine Free St. John's Wort
    Tea Bags

Manufacturer: Alvita Products, Inc; American Fork, UT; 801-756-9700
Form: 24 tea bags
Retail price: $3.79
Comments: Sold in health food stores.

OILS

Product Name: St. John's Wort Oil
Manufacturer: Mountain Rose Herbs; North San Juan, CA; 800-879-3337
Form: Oil for external use
No. of capsules/tablets per bottle: 2 oz., 4 oz.
Retail price: $6.95, $12.75
Comments: Product is for external use only. Available by mail order from the company.

Product Name: St. John's Wort Oil
Manufacturer: Herb Pharm; Williams, OR; 800-348-4372
Form: Oil for external use
Standardization: Not standardized
Amount per capsule/tablet (mg): Not known
Recommended daily dose: No recommended dose
Amount of liquid per bottle: 1 oz., 4 oz., 8 oz., 16 oz., 32 oz.
Retail price: $9.50, $36.10, $68.40, $129.20, $243.20
Comments: Herb is extracted in a base of olive oil and is applied to the skin. Available by

mail order from the company and in health food stores.

Product Name: Fresh St. John's Wort Flower Oil
Manufacturer: Gaia Herbs, Inc; Harvard, MA; 800-831-7780
Form: oil for external use
No. of capsules/tablets per bottle: 1 oz., 2 oz., 4 oz., 8 oz.
Retail price: $9.95, $18.95, $35.80, $67.75
Comments: Available in health food stores and by mail order from the company.

RAW HERB
Product Name: St. John's Wort Herb
Manufacturer: Mountain Rose Herbs; North San Juan, CA; 800-879-3337
Form: Dried herb, cut and sifted
No. of capsules/tablets per bottle: 4 oz., 8 oz., 16 oz.
Retail price: $4.75, $8.25, $16.00
Comments: Consists of the top part of the herb, which has been harvested and dried. Herb is certified organically grown. Can be used to make your own St. John's wort tea, tincture, or oil.

❧ CHAPTER 8 ❧

Defeating Depression
Through Diet

Although St. John's wort clearly works well on it own in defeating depression, you'll experience even better results if you make it a part of a comprehensive treatment plan that includes dietary changes. Good nutrition is important for all aspects of health, including mental health. And it's abundantly clear that for certain people, the symptoms of depression can be worsened by nutritional deficiencies.

Certain foods and dietary supplements can play major roles in helping to lift depression. Exposing yourself to these items usually won't involve radical changes in your diet—and the payoff in feeling better about yourself and about the world could be significant.

EMPHASIZE THE B VITAMINS

One of the most important things you can do to keep from getting depressed—or perhaps to help lift yourself out of a depression—is to make sure that you consume adequate amounts of the B vitamins—vitamin B_6, vitamin B_{12}, and folic acid.

In 1989, the medical establishment had so little regard for folic acid that the National Academy of Sciences recommended that the daily dose of this B vitamin should be reduced by half, from 400 micrograms per day to 200 micrograms. But over the past several years, the reputations of folic acid and the other two B vitamins has been greatly enhanced. Several recent studies have shown that these vitamins are vitally important—not only for good health in general but for our mental health in particular.

The brain requires folic acid, B_6 and B_{12} to manufacture its neurotransmitters, the chemicals responsible for sending messages throughout the brain. Depression is now recognized as resulting from inadequate levels of several of the neurotransitters—in particular serotonin, norepinephrine, and dopamine. (See Chapter Three for more information on depression's biochemical basis.)

Studies have shown that some people who suffer from severe depression or show signs of dementia have deficiencies of folic acid (also referred to as folate) or vitamin B_{12}. And it's known that correcting these deficiencies helps to dispel the depression and improve concentration and memory as well. Most importantly, you don't have to have a severe deficiency of the B vitamins to experience such adverse effects on mental health, since even a mild lack of the B vitamins can fog the mind.

In a recent study of 260 older people who showed no evidence of either illness or vitamin deficiency, the people with the lowest levels of vitamin B_{12} and folic acid in their blood scored significantly worse on tests of mental acuity than the rest of the group did. And in a second study, researchers at Tufts University artificially created a deficiency of vitamin B_6 by administering a specially restricted diet to older volunteers; the researchers then gave these volunteers modest levels of B_6 supplements and assessed their memory ability both while on the restricted diet and after the supplements were given. Memory was found to deteriorate steadily as vitamin B_6 levels fell, and it returned to normal after adequate levels were restored.

Unfortunately, many people consume inadequate amounts of two of these B vitamins, folic acid and vitamin B_6. (People who eat meat, fish, or dairy products generally don't have trouble getting enough vitamin B_{12}.) The average daily intake of folic acid by adults is about 285 micrograms (a microgram is a millionth of a gram), which is substantially less than the minimum of 400 micrograms previously recommended by the National

Academy of Sciences and currently listed by the federal government as the Recommended Daily Value. In addition, fewer than half of all Americans take in the recommended amount of vitamin B_6, which is two milligrams.

THE MANY BENEFITS OF FOLIC ACID AND B_6

Besides its usefulness in warding off depression, folic acid also plays several other crucial roles in maintaining good health. If women's diets are deficient in folic acid during the earliest days of their preganancy, their babies are at risk for developing spina bifida, a serious congenital disorder in which the spinal cord is not completely formed. Folic acid's importance in preventing spina bifida is the reason that, by 1998, the FDA will require that all enriched grain products such as bread, pasta, rice, flour, and cornmeal be fortified with folic acid.

Most recently, folic acid has received a great deal of publicity for its possible role in preventing heart disease by reducing levels of an amino acid in the blood called homocysteine. Elevated levels of homocysteine are believed to damage the lining of blood vessel walls and increase the risk for heart attacks. (There is also a weaker but still significant connection between shortages of vitamin B_6 or B_{12} and excessive homocysteine levels.)

Folic acid is found in green leafy vegetables such as lettuce, brussels sprouts, and spinach and in many fruits, including apples, oranges, and bananas. Most multiple vitamin preparations contain folic acid, and you can also buy it as a single-nutrient supplement.

Vitamin B_6 has a well-established role in improving serotonin function in the brain. Indeed, the body requires it to manufacture serotonin from the amino acid L-tryptophan (discussed below). But probably the most well-known use of vitamin B_6 is for easing the symptoms of premenstrual syndrome (PMS), a condition that occurs from seven to 14 days before a woman's period and can involve feelings of depression as well as mood swings, irritability, anxiety, headache, sugar cravings, and water retention.

Foods rich in vitamin B_6 include chicken, fish, avocados, potatoes, and watermelon; it also is contained in most multivitamins.

Several clinical studies have strengthened the notion that vitamin B_6 supplements may help against PMS. In one of the most impressive of these studies, 84 percent of women with PMS had a lower PMS symptom score during the vitamin B_6 treatment period than they did while taking a placebo. But if you're thinking about taking vitamin B_6 supplements for PMS, be careful not to take too much. Doses of more than 600 mg per day can cause a potentially serious nerve disorder called peripheral neuropathy, in which people experience numbness or tingling in their limbs. PMS can be successfully treated with much lower doses—as low as 50 mg per day.

In addition, for some women, oral contraceptives are known to cause depression that is linked to a deficiency of B_6. This problem can be corrected by treatment with a low dose of B_6.

Foods that are rich in vitamin B_6 include lean meats, chicken, fish, whole grains, bananas, avocados, watermelon, and potatoes. The Recommended Daily Value for vitamin B_6 is two milligrams. If you're in doubt about whether your diet is providing enough B_6, you can meet your needs for this vitamin by taking a daily multivitamin supplement.

As for vitamin B_{12}, the main sources in the human diet are meat, fish, and dairy products. People who consume these foods generally have little trouble obtaining enough vitamin B_{12} from their diet; as a result, it's uncommon for people to have a dietary deficiency of this vitamin. Even strict vegetarians, who avoid all meat and dairy products, may get enough B_{12} if they consume a lot of fortified cereals, tofu, soy beverages, or certain types of nutritional yeast. Check the label to see how much of this vitamin is in the foods you eat. Strict vegetarians who don't consume good sources of vitamin B_{12} should think about either eating cereals fortified with 100 percent of the Recommended Daily Value for this vitamin or taking a vitamin supplement.

The table below lists good food sources of folic acid, B_6, and B_{12}.

Table 3
Good Sources Of Vitamin B_6, B_{12}, and Folic Acid[1]

Food	Serving Size	Percent of U.S. Daily Value		
		Vitamin B_6	Vitamin B_{12}	Folic acid
MEAT AND FISH				
Alaskan king crab	3 oz	8	163	11
Atlantic mackerel	3 oz	20	268	0
Atlantic salmon	3 oz	40	43	6
Beef, sirloin	3 oz	19	41	2
Beef, top round	3 oz	24	35	3
Blue crab	3 oz	8	103	11
Bluefin tuna	3 oz	22	155	0
Bluefish	3 oz	20	88	0
Chicken breast, no skin	3 oz	26	5	1
Chicken liver	3 oz	25	275	164
Clams	3 oz	5	1,398	6

Food	Serving Size	Vitamin B_6	Vitamin B_{12}	Folic acid
Ground beef, extra lean	3 oz	14	37	2
Herring	3 oz	15	185	2
Leg of lamb	3 oz	6	37	4
Lobster	3 oz	3	44	2
Pork tenderloin	3 oz	22	14	1
Sardines	3 oz	7	127	3
Shrimp	3 oz	5	21	1
Turkey breast, no skin	3 oz	24	6	1
DAIRY				
Cottage cheese	½ cup	4	11	3
Milk, skim	1 cup	5	15	3
Yogurt, nonfat, plain	1 cup	7	25	7
FRUITS AND VEGETABLES[2]				
Asparagus	½ cup	5	0	24
Avocado, Florida	1	43	0	41
Banana	1	33	0	5
Broccoli	½ cup	6	0	12

Food	Serving Size	Vitamin B$_6$	Vitamin B$_{12}$	Folic acid
Brussels sprouts	½ cup	7	0	12
Escarole, raw	1 cup	1	0	18
Figs, dried	6	13	0	2
Green peas	½ cup	9	0	13
Orange juice, fresh	1 cup	5	0	19
Potato, baked, with skin	1 large	35	0	6
Romaine lettuce, raw	1 cup	1	0	19
Spinach	½ cup	11	0	33
Sweet potato, baked, peeled	1 medium	14	0	6
Watermelon	1 slice	35	0	3

LEGUMES

Food	Serving Size	Vitamin B$_6$	Vitamin B$_{12}$	Folic acid
Black-eyed peas	½ cup	4	0	45
Garbanzo beans	½ cup	6	0	35
Lentils	½ cup	9	0	45
Lima beans	½ cup	4	0	34

Food	Serving Size	Vitamin B$_6$	Vitamin B$_{12}$	Folic acid
Navy beans	½ cup	7	0	32
Pinto beans	½ cup	7	0	37
Red kidney beans	½ cup	5	0	29
GRAINS, NUTS, AND SEEDS				
Peanuts	¼ cup	5	0	11
Rice bran	1 tbsp	11	0	1
Sunflower seeds	¼ cup	14	0	20
Wheat germ, toasted	¼ cup	14	0	25
MISCELLANEOUS				
Brewer's yeast	1 tbsp	20	0	78
Soy drink	1 cup	8	13	6

[1]*Selected foods that contain at least 10 percent of the Recommended Daily Value of vitamin B$_6$, B$_{12}$ or folic acid (2 mg, 6 mcg, and 400 mcg, respectively).*
[2]*All vegetables cooked unless otherwise specified*
SOURCE: ESHA Research, Salem, OR

LET THE PYRAMID BE YOUR GUIDE

Probably the best—and simplest—way to make sure you get adequate amounts of the B vitamins

from your diet is to follow the diet widely recommended by public health authorities and summarized in the Food Guide Pyramid (pictured on
page 164). The U.S. Department of Agriculture
published it in 1992, to illustrate what it regarded
as a nutritious diet.

If you comply with the food-pyramid diet, the
generous quantities of fruits, vegetables, whole
grains, and beans that you'll consume should supply you with all of the folic acid you need. In addition, you'll also get more than enough vitamin
B_6 and—unless you're a strict vegetarian—enough
vitamin B_{12} as well.

By letting the food pyramid guide your eating
habits, you'll not only get enough of the B vitamins, but you'll also be consuming a good *overall*
diet for preventing depression and overcoming it
if it affects you. That's because of the eating style
that the pyramid espouses. Its broad bottom two
levels indicate that the bulk of our diet should consist of foods that are low in fat and high in fiber—
grains, beans, and cereals as well as vegetables
and fruits. On the other hand, the presence of fats,
oils, and sweets at the pyramid's apex indicates
that these foods should be eaten sparingly.

If we accept that old Latin saying *mens sano in
corpore sano*—a sound mind in a sound body—
then this is the best sort of diet for *overall* optimal
health, both physical and mental. Ultimately, the
pyramid can be viewed as a symbol for the following health-enhancing nutritional recommenda-

Food Guide Pyramid

A Guide to Daily Food Choices

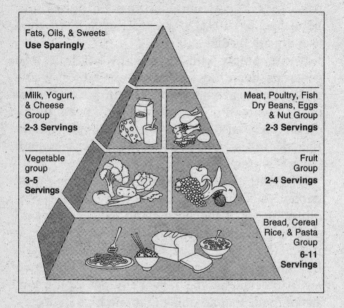

Fats, Oils, & Sweets
Use Sparingly

Milk, Yogurt,
& Cheese
Group
2-3 Servings

Meat, Poultry, Fish
Dry Beans, Eggs
& Nut Group
2-3 Servings

Vegetable
group
**3-5
Servings**

Fruit
Group
2-4 Servings

Bread, Cereal
Rice, & Pasta
Group
**6-11
Servings**

Use the Food Guide Pyramid to help you eat better every day . . . the Dietary Guidelines way. Start with plenty of Breads, Cereals, Rice, and Pasta; Vegetables; and Fruits. Add two to three servings from the Milk group and two to three servings from the Meat group. Each of these food groups provides some, but not all, of the nutrients you need. No one food group is more important than another—for good health you need them all. Go easy on fats, oils, and sweets, the foods in the small tip of the Pyramid.

tions for improving your physical and your mental health:

• *Cut down on your fat intake.* A federal survey released early in 1997 found that the percentage of overweight children, teenagers, and adults in the U.S. was "at an all-time high." Among adults, some 33 percent of men and 36 percent of women now qualify as overweight.

Being overweight can increase your risk for developing a slew of health problems including high blood pressure, an elevated blood cholesterol level, heart disease, several types of cancer, osteoarthritis, gallstones, and low-back problems. But in addition, being overweight can also increase your risk for developing emotional problems, including depression.

Low self-esteem, self-loathing, fatigue and lethargy, withdrawal from social activities are all symptoms of depression and can result from being overweight—or even more likely, from the frustration of our (often) unsuccessful efforts to lose the excess weight we've put on. And talk about frustration: Americans spend more than $10 billion a year on commercial weight-loss programs; yet studies show that fewer than one in seven so-called successful graduates of these weight-loss programs are able to maintain significant weight loss a year later. If you are overweight, cutting down on fat is one of the most important things you can do to shed the pounds that are weighing you down both physically and emotionally.

As a nation, we eat too much fat. Federal recommendations suggest that people should restrict the percentage of their calories from fat to 30 percent—and many scientists believe that fat intake should ideally be much lower, with no more than 15 or 20 percent of calories from fat. Clearly we have a long way to go, since the average American gets 36 percent of their calories from fat.

• *Favor fiber.* Perhaps the best way of all for you to lower the amount of fat in your diet is to eat more foods that are high in fiber. The high-fiber foods emphasized in the food pyramid—vegetables, fruits, grains, and beans—also tend to be low in both calories and fat. Switching from a typical American diet to one rich in these foods should definitely help you to lose more weight—or keep you from becoming overweight in the first place. Several clinical trials comparing similar weight-loss regimens have shown that adding fiber to your diet can help you lose an average of four additional pounds over a two- to three-month period.

And even if you don't lose weight on a diet rich in fiber, this diet will improve your overall health in other important ways. A substantial body of research shows that a high-fiber diet helps to reduce heart disease risk by lowering cholesterol levels; lowers the risk for diabetes; helps to prevent colon cancer; may help to prevent breast cancer; and may reduce the risk for developing high blood pressure.

If you're like many people, your fiber intake is less than optimal. Half of all Americans consume less than 14 grams of fiber a day, while health experts typically recommend that healthy adults should consume between 20 and 35 grams of fiber daily. But by following the food pyramid, you can significantly increase your fiber intake.

The pyramid's foundation consists of six to 11 servings per day of grains—bread, cereal, rice, and pasta. All of these foods are potentially high in fiber if you choose whole-grain products. Stick with unrefined items such as whole-grain breads and whole-wheat pasta, brown rice, and cereals such as shredded wheat and bran flakes. You will also get plentiful amounts of fiber from the pyramid's next level, which provides three to five servings per day of vegetables and two to four servings of fruit.

If you've resolved to increase your intake of fiber, try not to go overboard. Consuming a lot more than the recommended maximum of 35 grams of fiber per day can interfere with the body's absorption of calcium, iron, zinc, and other nutrients. Be careful to boost your fiber intake gradually, since doing it too fast can cause gas, bloating, cramping, or diarrhea.

• *Eat five or more servings of fruit and vegetables per day.* The federal food pyramid calls for "Five a Day," or five servings daily of some combination of fruits and vegetables. We've noted that fruit and vegetables can help you increase your fiber intake, but in addition they provide you with antioxidants, the chemicals that can help to protect against a wide range of chronic diseases associated with aging, including heart disease, several types of cancer, and osteoarthritis. We need antioxidants to combat chemicals known as free radicals, which are now suspected of playing a major role in causing these chronic diseases.

The free radicals damage cell membranes, DNA, and proteins throughout the body. Recent research shows that diets high in antioxidants help protect people against the damage that these free radicals cause—damage implicated in causing a number of chronic diseases including several types of cancer, arthritis, and Alzheimer's disease. It's all too clear that the emotional burden of chronic diseases, which so often afflict the elderly, helps to account for their increased susceptibility to depression. By helping to prevent these chronic diseases, a diet rich in antioxidants can help to ward off depression as well.

While the food pyramid's recommendation of five servings of fruits and vegetables daily is a worthy goal, it actually may not be sufficient. Many nutrition experts believe that we should consume even more—at least seven servings of produce daily. Unfortunately, only one in five Americans eats five or more daily servings of fruits and vegetables, and a mere one in 20 of us consumes seven servings.

L-TRYPTOPHAN: GONE BUT NOT FORGOTTEN

The amino acid L-tryptophan is important to good mental health because it is the main building block for the body's production of serotonin, the neurotransmitter that is now recognized as so important in determining whether people become depressed.

L-trytophan is one of the 23 essential amino acids that are the building blocks of serotonin and all other proteins. "Essential" means that the body cannot synthesize L-tryptophan from other substances, but instead it must be obtained directly from the diet.

For more than 30 years, Americans used L-tryptophan supplements for insomnia and also for depression. During that time, L-tryptophan was notable for causing only mild side effects such as dizziness, nausea, and headache. But in 1989, a number of people taking L-tryptophan went to their doctors and to emergency rooms with alarming symptoms—high fever, weakness, swelling of the arms and legs, shortness of breath, and severe muscle and joint pain. As a result, health food store owners and other retailers removed L-tryptophan from their shelves.

Ultimately, 38 L-tryptophan users died and another 1,500 people were seriously injured from this cluster of symptoms, which was later named eosinophilia myalgia syndrome (EMS). Virtually all of these deaths and illnesses were linked to L-tryptophan obtained from one of the six Japanese companies that supplied L-tryptophan to the United States. This company, Showa Denko, had changed the way it made L-tryptophan—a change that apparently introduced a toxic contaminant that was responsible for the EMS.

The cause of these tragic deaths and illnesses can almost certainly be attributed to the contaminant in Showa Denko's L-tryptophan and not to L-tryptophan in general. Nevertheless, the FDA has still not allowed L-tryptophan back on store shelves.

As it turns out, L-tryptophan does help to promote sleep—as little as one gram is effective. But although it's the body's main building block for making serotonin, L-tryptophan by itself does not appear to work in alleviating depression. Nevertheless, you should make sure that your diet includes foods that are good sources of L-tryptophan: the amount of serotonin in your brain depends on the level of L-tryptophan that is in your blood and how much of it crosses the blood-brain barrier and enters the brain.

Examples of foods rich in L-tryptophan include turkey, chicken, fish, cooked dried beans and peas, peanut butter, Brewer's yeast, nuts, and soybeans. One possible complication: As it is being taken up from the blood and passed into the brain, L-tryptophan is part of a transport system in which it competes with several other amino acids including isoleucine, valine, tyrosine and phenylalanine. Since the amount of these other amino acids in foods generally exceeds the amount of L-tryptophan, a protein-rich meal by itself will result in relatively little L-tryptophan being absorbed into the brain.

THE CARBOHYDRATE CONNECTION

There *is* a good way to to enhance the brain's absorption of L-tryptophan from the blood-stream—and that's to eat a carbohydrate-rich meal or snack. The food can be a complex carbohydrate such as bread, grain, rice or pasta, or it can consist of simple carbohydrates such as table sugar or fruits and vegetables, which also contain sugars.

Whatever the carbohydrate you eat, it triggers the pancreas to release insulin, the hormone that regulates the amount of sugar in the bloodstream. But in addition, insulin prompts the body's tissues to take up the amino acids that are circulating in the blood and to use them for building proteins. This has the effect of lowering the levels of amino acids available to travel across the blood-brain barrier—and leaves L-tryptophan present in relatively higher amounts for making that trip compared with its amino acid competitors. Thanks to this boost from carboyhdrates, L-tryptophan can now start to arrive in higher amounts in the brain, where it is used to produce serotonin.

To get the most out of this mood-food connection, proper timing of your carbohydrate meal is essential. (When you eat foods rich in L-tryptophan is less important, since the amount of L-tryptophan in the blood remains relatively stable throughout the day.) Experiments with laboratory animals have provided some useful findings on how carbohydrates interact with L-tryptophan to boost brain serotonin levels. Here is what is known so far:

• If your first meal of the day contains mostly carbohydrates and very little protein (a buttered bagel, orange juice, and sugar-sweetened coffee, for example), you'll experience a sharp increase in brain serotonin about two or three hours later.

• No such increase in serotonin will occur if your first meal of the day is mainly protein (eggs and bacon, for example).

• A combined protein-carbohydrate meal (bacon, eggs, toast and orange juice) will also fail to raise brain serotonin levels. That's because digestion of all that protein will flood the bloodstream with many different amino acids, effectively overwhelming the L-tryptophan that may be present.

• Eating carbohydrates soon after you have a protein or a mixed protein-carbohydrate meal also has little effect on brain serotonin levels.

The conclusion from all the studies to date that have looked at interactions between carbohydrate and L-tryptophan: You'll need a relatively pure carbohydrate meal or snack on an empty stomach to attain the mood-lifting effect of increased brain serotonin production.

SUCCUMB TO CARBOHYDRATE CRAVINGS?

It is now known that carbohydrate meals can also improve mood by boosting brain serotonin levels directly—without having to act through L-tryptophan. Could it be, as some experts have theorized, that people with low serotonin levels are "drawn to" carbohydrate-rich food, in much the same way that deer and other animals will go to great lengths to obtain the tiny amount of salt they need to survive? There is some suggestive evidence in favor of this notion. For example, many women who are experiencing the symptoms of PMS have a craving for carbohydrate-rich food; their craving could actually be their bodies' way of relieving PMS symptoms by raising their serotonin levels.

The theory was bolstered recently by a study in which women with PMS were asked to eat a carbohydrate-rich (protein-poor) dinner during the late luteal phase of their menstrual cycle (i.e., a few days before their period was expected). After eating the carbohydrate-rich meal, the women noticed a significant improvement in their PMS symptoms. It has also been noticed that PMS sufferers tend to reduce their carbohydrate consumption if they are treated with Prozac or other SSRI antidepressants that boost serotonin levels.

A similar craving occurs in people suffering from seasonal affective disorder: About two-thirds of people with SAD report that they have an increased appetite for carbohydrates during the winter months, with a preference for starches such as pasta, bread, potatoes, rice, and corn. These "heavy" carbohydrate foods apparently help to brighten their mood and reduce their fatigue; conversely, their intake of carbohydrates falls off during the summer or when they are given L-tryptophan supplements or antidepressants such as Prozac.

Can carbohydrate-rich food help your mood? That question hasn't been answered conclusively, but this is certainly one psychological experiment that you can perform on yourself without having to worry about adverse effects. But while you're at it, try to emphasize complex carbohydrate foods such as bagels, pasta with tomato sauce, or whole-grain breads. These foods are much healthier than high-fat carbohydrates such as potato chips or french fries.

AVOID ALCOHOL

If you're feeling depressed, the last thing you should do is ingest a depressant chemical. Yet that's what alcohol is—a chemical whose principal effect is to depress the central nervous system.

Unfortunately, alcohol and depression often go together, a phenomenon known as co-morbidity.

On the one hand, studies show that from 16 to 59 percent of alcoholics (who represent from five to 10 percent of the U.S. population) become depressed. Conversely, depressed people often resort to alcohol as a way to lift their spirits. One study found that serious depression was a problem in 70 percent of patients with prolonged heavy drinking. And according to population studies carried out by the National Institute of Mental Health, half of women alcoholics are seriously depressed—and two-thirds of them were depressed *before* they began abusing alcohol.

So if you're depressed, you should realize that you're at risk for becoming addicted to alcohol. And if you're an alcoholic, depression is one of the many possible adverse consequences that are possible.

CAFFEINE: GOOD OR BAD?

Caffeine, the main active ingredient in coffee, has been used for centuries as a mild central nervous system stimulant. It has quite a widespread stimulating effect, affecting the heart, lungs, stomach (by increasing the production of stomach acids), and other organs, as well as the muscles.

Since it does have a stimulating effect, caffeine can help to elevate the mood of certain depressed people. A seventeenth-century paean to coffee noted that the beverage "quickeneth the spirits" and "maketh the heart lightsom"—effects that were no doubt due to caffeine, which probaby ranks as America's favorite drug. Recently, caffeine's mood-boosting effects have been borne out by several studies.

In one of those studies, researchers at Johns Hopkins University gave nine coffee drinkers a pill that contained either caffeine or a placebo; the volunteers, who didn't know which pill they were receiving on which day, took the pill they were given for 40 days in a row. They reported feeling more awake, energetic, self-confident, and friendly when they were given the caffeine rather than the dummy pill. These, of course, are improvements in mood that could especially benefit people who are feeling depressed.

Caffeine also exerts antidepressive effects by fighting drowsiness, fatigue, and boredom. For example, it can improve performance on routine and somewhat boring tasks such as typing, filing, or simple bookkeeping and help you stay alert during prolonged and potentially sleep-inducing tasks such as driving.

But while consuming moderate amounts of caffeine can clearly improve your mood and performance, drinking too much can overstimulate the nerves and provoke several of the symptoms of depression, including anxiety, restlessness, and irritability; in addition, there may be trembling of the hands and difficulty falling asleep. Even more troubling effects, including depression, can occur when people develop a dependency on caffeine—

and it doesn't take much caffeine to make people become dependent on it.

In one study in which coffee-drinking volunteers were asked to stop drinking coffee for a while, fully half the volunteers who ordinarily drank just one to three cups of coffee a day developed headaches—the main symptom of caffeine withdrawal. About 10 percent became depressed, anxious or fatigued, and some of them reported experiencing flulike symptoms, nausea, and even vomiting. Some even felt sick enough to call their doctors. Other studies have found a definite link between caffeine and depression.

For example, in one study of healthy college students, moderate and high quantity coffee drinkers scored higher on a depression scale than did light coffee users. Other studies have found that depressed patients tend to consume large amounts of coffee—and that there is a correlation between coffee consumption and depression: The more coffee people drank, the more likely they were to be severely depressed. (But these studies don't necessarily prove that caffeine plays a role in causing or aggravating depression; they could merely indicate that depressed people seek out coffee as a way to self-medicate.)

Probably the main depression threat posed by coffee (or other caffeinated liquids such as colas) is to heavy drinkers of those beverages who try to stop their habit. Such people may become depressed or experience other symptoms of caffeine withdrawal including fatigue, headache, and irritability. The best way to avoid depression and the other symptoms of caffeine withdrawal is to wean yourself gradually from coffee rather than stopping all at once.

And keep in mind that coffee is not the only liquid that can leave you vulnerable to depression and other symptoms of caffeine withdrawal. Two to four cans of caffeinated soda, or two to four cups of tea, can provide as much caffeine as a cup or two of regular coffee; for regular soda drinkers, that's enough to provoke symptoms if you skip taking the beverage for as little as half a day.

EAT MORE FISH

In his classic book *The Anatomy of Melancholy*, published in 1652, Robert Burton recommended a low-fat diet that included fish as a treatment for "melancholy," or what we now refer to as depression. It now seems apparent that Burton was on to something.

Fish—especially fatty, cold-water ones such as mackerel and herring—are rich in omega-3 polyunsaturated fatty acids. In fact, fish are our main dietary source of omega-3. Only relatively recently have scientists appreciated that these omega-3 fatty acids are crucial to the normal functioning of the body.

The omega-3's first received publicity in the 1980's, because of studies carried on Greenland Eskimos. Despite consuming a high-fat diet due to living mainly on fatty fish, the Eskimos were found to have a remarkably low incidence of heart disease. Later studies showed that when omega-3 fatty acids are added to the western diet, they cause a number of metabolic changes.

Fish oil can help reduce inflammation, and several clinical studies have shown that fish oil supplements may offer modest benefits in easing the symptoms of arthritis. Also, the omega-3 from fish are now recognized as important nutrients for vision, immune function, and for possible protection against several types of cancer. The omega-3's are also important in nerve function, and now it appears that they may play an important role in preventing and treating depression.

When we swallow fats of any kinds, we incorporate their fatty acids into the cell membranes of all the cells in our bodies, including our nerve cells. Whether a cell membrane is "rich" in one kind of fatty acid or another has a big effect on the physiological properties of that membrane—which, in turn, has a major influence on the functioning of the cell itself. As a result, cells with membranes that are rich in omega-3's) function differently from cells whose membranes mainly contain the other kind of fatty acids, the omega-6's. (The omega-6 fatty acids, which come mainly from vegetable oils and meats, are the predominant fatty acid in Western diets.)

Recently, a study published in the *American Journal of Clinical Nutrition* offered provocative evidence that decreased omega-3 consumption over the past century may be responsible for the increasing rates of depression over that time. The study, written by two researchers at the National Institute of Alcohol Abuse and Alcoholism, postulates that adequate amounts of omega-3 polyunsaturated fatty acids in the diet may reduce the development of depression, just as they may help in reducing coronary artery disease. The authors make the following points:

• Societies consuming large amounts of fish and omega-3 fatty acids appear to have lower rates of major depression. In Japan, for example, where fish consumption is high, rates of depression are estimated at 0.35 percent for men and 0.46 percent for women. By comparison, a recent national survey of depression in three United States cities found rates for depression that were on the order of 10 times greater.

• Several studies have shown that chronic alcoholism strips omega-3 from the membranes of nerve cells, which may contribute to the depressive symptoms that so often affect alcoholics.

• Pregnancy depletes the level of omega-3 fatty acids in the prospective mother's bloodstream, presumably because these nutrients are vital to the developing fetus's nervous system. This depletion of omega-3 in a mother's blood may be one of the complex factors responsible for postpartum depression, as well as the increased risk of depression faced by women of childbearing age.

• The current view of depression is that it results from the reduced functioning of serotonin, norepinephrine and other neurotransmitters in the brain. Data suggest that polyunsaturated fatty acids in the diet may affect the function of neurotransmitters—the amount produced, their degradation, their reuptake, and how effectively neurotransmitters bind to receptors.

Although the role of omega-3 fatty acids in causing depression must still be confirmed by further studies, it's abundantly clear that fish oil and its omega-3 fatty acids have a number of positive impacts on physical health. So it makes sense to substitute fish for at least some of the meat and dairy foods you eat, and many health professionals now advocate eating three or more fish meals per week.

The table below lists a variety of fish and the amounts of omega-3 fatty acids, saturated fat, and total fat that they contain. Although eating fish is the natural way to gain the benefits of the omega-3, fish oil supplements such as MaxEPA and SuperEPA are alternative ways to add omega-3 to your diet. (For comparison, one 1,000-mg fish-oil capsule generally contains 0.3 to 0.5 grams of omega-3 fatty acids.)

Table 4
Fat content of selected seafood

Food (3 oz)	Omega-3 fatty acids (g)	Saturated fat (g)	Total fat (g)	Calories
Atlantic salmon	1.9	1.1	6.9	155
Herring	1.8	2.2	9.8	172
Whitefish	1.6	1.0	6.4	146
Bluefin tuna	1.3	1.4	5.3	156
Sardines, canned in oil	1.3	1.3	9.7	177
Mackerel	1.1	3.6	15.2	223
Sockeye salmon	1.1	1.6	9.3	184
Rainbow trout	1.0	1.4	5.0	128
Swordfish	0.9	1.2	4.4	132
Bluefish	0.8	1.0	4.6	135
Scallops	0.8	0.6	3.4	113
Bass, freshwater	0.8	0.9	4.0	124
Blue mussels, steamed (7)	0.7	0.7	3.8	146
Catfish	0.5	1.0	5.0	120

Food (3 oz)	Omega-3 fatty acids (g)	Saturated fat (g)	Total fat (g)	Calories
Halibut	0.5	0.4	2.5	119
Pollock	0.5	0.1	1.0	100
Sole/ flounder	0.4	0.3	1.3	100
Ocean perch	0.4	0.3	1.8	103
Chinook salmon/ lox, smoked	0.4	0.8	3.7	99
Alaskan king crab, steamed	0.4	0.1	1.3	82
Shrimp, steamed (15 med)	0.3	0.2	0.9	84
Clams, steamed (12 small)	0.2	0.2	1.7	126
Pacific cod	0.2	0.1	0.7	99
Tuna, canned in water	0.2	0.2	0.7	99
Haddock	0.2	0.1	0.8	95

❖ CHAPTER 9 ❖

Coping with Depression
Through Lifestyle Changes

The current emphasis on neurotransmitters in depression obscures an important fact: Depression results from a complex interplay of many factors—not only the biochemistry of your brain but also the way you've lived your life: your upbringing, what you eat and drink, whether you have a support network, and how susceptible you are to stress.

All of these lifestyle influences can have a major impact—for good or for ill—on whether or not you become depressed and how successfully you cope with your depression. This chapter will offer some recommendations concerning the most important of these lifestyle factors—the ones to avoid as well as well as those that are helpful.

DON'T ABUSE ALCOHOL

As noted in the previous chapter, many people who abuse alcohol become depressed. And, conversely, depressed people often resort to alcohol in a misguided attempt to lift their spirits—misguided because alcohol is a powerful central nervous system depressant, which is the last thing you need if you're battling depression.

AVOID ILLICIT DRUGS

Illicit drugs such as cocaine or speed may initially cause euphoria but all too often lead to a crash that can involve depression or even more serious consequences.

BE WARY OF CERTAIN MEDICATIONS

Quite a long list of drugs now being sold can actually cause depression. Among these are drugs for treating high blood pressure, such as reserpine, methyldopa (Aldomet), clonidine (Catepres) and propranolol (Inderal); drugs such as L-dopa and bromocriptine that are used for treating Parkinson's disease; diet pills; oral contraceptives; drugs for treating arthritis, including indomethacin (Indocin) and corticosteroids; and drugs used in hormone replacement therapy, including estrogen and progesterone.

DON'T SMOKE

It's advice that has been given so many times over so many years it may have lost the power to influence anyone—especially considering that one out of every four adult Americans still smokes. But in addition to the terrible toll that smoking can have on physical health, it is also a leading contributor to depression.

Many smokers claim that cigarettes increase their alertness and help them to think more clearly—and there is some evidence for that. But over the long term, cigarette smoking's main effect on the mind is to depress it.

The so-called blood-brain barrier, which protects the brain from many potentially toxic substances that we ingest or inhale, provides no defense against nicotine, the drug responsible for dependence on tobacco and that also acts as a stimulant. Within 10 seconds of that first drag, nicotine slips through the blood-brain barrier and latches onto receptors that the neurotransmitter acetylcholine normally fits into when it transmits messages to adjacent cells.

But nicotine has a different effect on nerve cells, causing them to release two other neurotransmitters, noradrenaline and dopamine, which act as stimulants. This produces a short-lived lift—

smoking increases alertness, thinking ability, and the ability to perform although fatigued—but causes longer-term damage to the psyche: Smokers are more likely to be depressed than nonsmokers; people who are depressed are more likely to smoke; smokers with a history of depression have more severe psychological symptoms than nonsmokers; and depressed smokers have a tougher time coping with their depression if they try to stop smoking.

Important differences also exist between depressed and nondepressed smokers, with depressed smokers more likely to experience withdrawal symptoms when they try to quit. Depressed smokers are less likely to be successful at quitting and more likely to relapse. In fact, in one large study of smoking cessation, depression was the most significant reason for relapse. The authors of this study estimated that from 30 to 40 percent of people who begin smoking-cessation programs are depressed—three times higher than the incidence of depression in nonsmokers.

If you smoke, do your best to quit—not only because you're at risk for depression but because of all the ways that smoking can damage health. If you're already a depressed smoker and you want to quit your habit, try to find a smoking-cessation program that is tailored to the needs of depressed smokers. When it comes to helping depressed smokers quit their habit, researchers have found that antidepressant medication, psychological support, and nicotine-replacement therapy are all useful in achieving success.

EMPHASIZE FULFILLING PERSONAL RELATIONSHIPS

For people who want to overcome depression—or avoid becoming depressed in the first place—social interaction is extremely important. Try to spend time with people you care about, especially those friends or family members who are supportive rather than critical of you. Aside from the peace of mind that social interaction can produce, studies show that social contact has definite—and positive—physiological effects. It can lower pulse rate and blood pressure, enhance the immune system and boost the production of endorphins, those neurochemicals that make us feel better.

CONSIDER A SUPPORT GROUP

Back in the 1930's, two acquaintances struggling with alcoholism—a businessman and a physician—came to the realization that they could stay sober by talking to each other. They began talking to other alcoholics as well and eventually formed the first support group—Alcoholics Anonymous, or AA.

The success of AA has inspired the creation of support groups for people with scores of different health problems, including depression. Many people with depression—or, for that matter, *any* health problem—regard participating in a support group or self-help group to be an integral part of their recovery. In a typical support group, five to 10 people with the same problem meet each week to offer encouragement and to share their experiences in coping with a difficult situation. At support group meetings, the idea is not to wallow in self-pity but rather to search for solutions to problems. Participation is almost always free of charge.

The support group sessions are run by the members themselves. In some support groups, family members are invited to attend all or some of the meetings. In addition, some support groups invite guest experts to speak; in the case of a depression group, this might be a local therapist who specializes in treating the problem. In Chapter Twelve, we tell you who you can contact to find out about support groups in your area.

OPTING FOR PSYCHOTHERAPY

For people who are depressed, social support can be extremely valuable in coping with the problem of depression and eventually overcoming it. And for many people who suffer from mild depression, the support provided by family or friends can provide all the help that is needed. But sometimes professional help may be required, particularly if a person is despondent or is having trouble coping with life.

People suffering from depression may be able to benefit from one of several kinds of psychotherapies that are offered by a variety of different mental health professionals: psychiatrists, psychologists, social workers, marriage and family therapists, and psychiatric nurses.

For readers of this book in particular, the "talk therapies" offered by these professionals may have special appeal, since talking is clearly a more natural approach to treating depression than taking synthetic antidepressant medications. But you should be aware that major depression is now viewed as a *biological* illness, resulting from abnormally low levels of neurotransmitters in the brain. While some people can definitely benefit from talk therapies, others will need antidepressant medications—including possibly St. John's wort—to help correct their neurotransmitter imbalance and overcome their depression. In fact, among psychiatrists who treat depressed patients, many believe they'd be committing malpractice if they didn't offer antidepressant medication to their severely depressed patients.

CHOOSING A THERAPIST AND A THERAPY

Anyone considering treatment for depression has a wide choice of therapies and practitioners. When choosing a therapist, you should make sure that the person is truly qualified to provide the high-quality care that you deserve. Unfortunately, anyone can legally call themselves a psychotherapist—regardless of whether that person has received the training and supervision necessary to practice in a competent way. If possible, look for someone who is licensed or certified in the following areas:

Psychiatrists are physicians who have completed medical school and a one-year internship, followed by three years of residency training in psychiatry. All psychiatrists are trained in psychiatric diagnosis and in pharmacotherapy—the use of antidepressants and other drugs for treating emotional problems. Psychiatrists are the only therapists who have the authority to prescribe antidepressant drugs.

Psychoanalysts may have a professional degree in one of a number of areas—psychiatry, psychology, or social work. In addition, they have had at least two years of extensive supervised training at a psychoanalytic institute.

Psychologists who have the credentials Ph.D., Ed.D., or Psy.D. are licensed professional counselors who have doctoral-level training, which usually includes a year of clinical internship in a mental health facility and a year of supervised postdoctoral experience.

Social workers usually get their training in a two-year master's degree program that involves fieldwork in a wide range of settings, including mental health settings. Those social workers who continue on to seek state certification or licensing as *clinical* social workers require two years of supervised postgraduate experience and must pass a statewide examination.

Family and marriage therapists may have earned a master's or doctoral degree from an accredited graduate training program in the field, or they have received another professional degree with supervised experience in the specialty.

Psychiatric nurses are registered nurses (R.N.s) who work in mental-health settings. Often they are part of a therapeutic team that may include psychiatrists and psychologists. Advanced practice nurses have a master's degree and can provide psychotherapy.

The basic types of therapies that are used in treating depression are the following:

Psychodynamic therapy. This form of therapy is based on the premise that unconscious psychological conflicts—for example, feeling angry while at the same time believing that you should always be kind and loving—are the source of the patient's problem. Some of these conflicts may be traceable to early childhood and may arise from difficult relationships between parent and child. In psychodynamic therapy, the goal is to bring those conflicts into the open where they can be discussed and, hopefully resolved, thereby resulting in successful treatment.

The problem with psychodynamic therapy is that it's open-ended—lasting for years in some cases—and therefore can be quite expensive.

More recently, researchers have developed abbreviated, time-limited therapies that largely ignore childhood traumas and instead focus on present-day concerns.

Two of these short-term therapies in particular—*cognitive therapy* and *interpersonal therapy*—seem to offer effective alternatives to longer-term treatment, especially for people with milder forms of depression. These therapies generally last for 10 to 20 sessions over several months and focus on the here and now rather than on problems in the past, such as childhood traumas. During that time, the patient and therapist discuss specific problems involved in causing and perpetuating the depression.

Cognitive therapy. This form of therapy was developed by Dr. Aaron Beck, a psychiatrist at the University of Pennsylvania School of Medicine. In cognitive therapy, depression is seen as resulting from a depressed person's negative and distorted views of themselves and the world around them—a pessimistic stance that they may have learned as children or as adolescents without ever realizing it. Negative thinking has long been recognized as a sign of depression, but Beck contends that it is the actual cause.

In cognitive therapy, the therapist tries to get the patient to focus on their negative "cognitions," or thoughts, and to recognize the link between their negative way of thinking and the depression they're feeling. The idea is to get patients to be aware of situations where they automatically think negatively and to ask themselves if such thoughts are warranted by the evidence. Once the patient recognizes that their negative thinking is distorted thinking, then, hopefully, they'll start to view the world in a more positive way.

While cognitive therapy does not appear to help when people are severely depressed, several clinical studies have now found it to be effective in treating about 70 percent of people with mild to moderately severe depression. In addition, for these milder cases of depression, cognitive therapy has been found to be as effective as antidepressant medication.

Interpersonal therapy. This type of therapy, which is approximately equal to cognitive therapy in its effectiveness against depression, was developed by Gerald Klerman, M.D., a psychiatrist at Harvard University and Myrna Weissman, Ph.D., a psychologist and depression researcher at Columbia University's New York State Psychiatric Institute. Interpersonal therapy focuses on getting depressed people to identify the problems they have in their relationships with others—particularly problems that may have contributed to their depressed mood—and work to resolve those problems by relating better to other people.

In interpersonal therapy, patients learn to understand that positive relationships with others are crucial to mental health. They also learn skills to help them communicate better and otherwise function more effectively in relationships.

This type of therapy is best suited to those people whose relationship problems are either the cause or the result of their depressed mood. But for suitable candidates, cognitive therapy can definitely help. In a 1989 study sponsored by the National Institute of Mental Health, up to 69 percent of patients who completed a four-month course of interpersonal therapy no longer experienced depressive symptoms and functioned more effectively at home and at work.

Some mildly depressed people will do better with psychotherapy than with any medication—and that includes St. John's wort as well as the synthetic antidepressants. But psychotherapy usually isn't a sufficient treatment for people troubled by severe depression. For these people, the most effective treatment may be a combination of psychotherapy and antidepressant medication. Certainly, people whose depression fails to respond to psychotherapy should be evaluated by a specialist—preferably a psychiatrist—to learn if they are a candidate for medication.

DE-STRESS YOURSELF

Stress is one of the most important factors involved in depression. By making changes in your lifestyle, you can help minimize stress's adverse impact on your mind and body. Such stress-defying changes can help you to overcome depression or even keep it from occurring.

When it comes to stress and depression, it's not

always easy to know which one causes the other. Depressed people often exhibit anxiety, agitation, and other signs of stress. And equally important, stress itself can clearly play a role in causing depression.

Stress can be thought of as something that interferes with a person's mental or physical well-being. Stressors—those things that cause us stress—can include a wide range of physical and emotional events such as physical violence, internal conflicts like as guilt, and significant life events, including the death of a friend or loved one, the birth of a baby, the loss of a job, or a divorce.

Increasingly, research is showing that the amount of stress that people confront is not as important as their capacity to handle it: Some people simply have a greater tolerance for negative events than others do. Everyone, however, has a "breaking point" for stress, the point at which stress begins to overwhelm a person's ability to absorb it and begins to affect his body in ways that can be detrimental.

First the voluntary nervous system, which responds to sensory input and controls our voluntary movements, sends messages to your muscles so that you're prepared for that most primitive of responses, the fight-or-flight response. Then the autonomic nervous system, which controls involuntary bodily functions, prepares your muscles for action by sending extra blood to them while at the same time it diverts blood from other bodily functions such as digestion. Finally, the neuroendocrine system releases two hormones—adrenaline, the hormone that primes the body for action, and cortisol, a hormone that magnifies and extends adrenaline's effects.

This stress-induced surge of hormones and other chemicals speeds up the heart rate, raises blood pressure, and revs up the body's metabolism—all of which may have helped our prehistoric ancestors survive in dangerous situations. But constant exposure to stress leaves our bodies unable to recover, wearing us down and leading to serious physical and mental symptoms—headache, backache, anxiety, insomnia, arthritis, gastrointestinal upset, skin disorders, weight loss, weight gain, anxiety, heart palpitations, drug and alcohol abuse and, finally, depression.

Many cases of depression can be traced to a stressful event. Through a complex interaction involving stress, a person's underlying genetic susceptibility to depression, and neurotransmitters in the brain, a person becomes enveloped by the feelings of sadness, guilt, anxiety, loss of interest in usual activities, and the other symptoms that characterize depression.

In today's world, stress is unavoidable. But since we must face it, we have to learn to deal with stress if we're to keep it from afflicting us with depression and other emotional and physical ills. Here are some changes you can make in your life that can help you to handle stress better.

PRACTICE A RELAXATION TECHNIQUE

All of the numerous relaxation techniques have the same basic aim in common: to help you release muscle tension and achieve a state of mental calm. These techniques are particularly helpful for relieving stress resulting from personal problems, difficulties on the job, or any other reason. Some of the basic relaxation techniques include active and passive relaxations, biofeedback, and imagery.

Active relaxation. This involves tensing and then relaxing your entire body, usually starting with your feet and then slowly moving up the body, one area at at time, until you finally tense and relax the muscles in your neck and head. Active relaxation makes you aware of the contrast between muscles that are tense and muscles that are relaxed. The aim is for the technique to "enlighten" your muscles, helping them to realize that being relaxed feels much better than being tense.

Passive relaxation. Meditation is perhaps the best example of passive relaxation. It involves clearing the mind of distractions and focusing on a single phrase or word and then repeating it over and over. Concentrating in this way helps to keep thoughts of pain or stress from entering your consciousness. It's not uncommon for such unwanted thoughts to intrude during meditation; don't let that bother you, instead simply refocus on the phrase or word that you have been repeating.

While meditating, you should also concentrate on controlling your breathing, keeping in mind that hyperventilation—breathing that is rapid and shallow—can be counterproductive by causing or worsening stress. Although meditation need not take up a lot of time—even meditating for a single minute can slow your heartbeat and lower your blood pressure—you generally achieve deeper relaxation during longer sessions of 15 minutes or more.

If thinking peaceful thoughts or focusing on your breathing sounds too mystical for you, try a more conventional form of passive relaxation such as listening to music. Choose whatever soothes your psyche, whether it's The Rolling Stones or Gregorian chants. Audiotapes are also available and can guide you through the process of relaxing.

Biofeedback. In this relaxation technique, you get "feedback" on a normally unconscious function of the body, such as your blood pressure, so that you can ultimately gain control over it—and improve your health by doing so. Such training is especially helpful for warding off stress as well as anxiety.

At the start of a biofeedback session, special monitoring devices are attached to your body to measure your heart rate, blood pressure, skin temperature, muscle tension, or other bodily activity of which you're not normally aware. Changes in the measuring signals—flashing lights, fluctuating needles, or a sound that varies in tone—will then provide you with information (feedback) on how your blood pressure or other bodily functions are changing.

After awhile, you'll learn to change the signal by consciously controlling the body function being measured—blood pressure, heart rate, brain waves, etc. With practice, you become aware of how you feel whenever there is a change in the signal—and you'll eventually be able to self-regulate a body function without being attached to the monitoring device. For example, you'll be able to lower your heart rate or blood pressure, which means that you'll have taught yourself how to relax. Once you master biofeedback, you can put it into practice when you're confronted with stressful situations.

Imagery. In this relaxation technique, you use your imagination to conjure up particular experiences or scenes that produce feelings of peace or comfort within you. The aim is to become so absorbed in thinking about colors, sounds, or smells of the scene you're imagining that these positive feelings distract you from the anxiety or stress that you're under.

ENGAGE IN EXERCISE

Whether you're someone who is seriously depressed or a person who just occasionally experiences the blues, getting into the exercise habit can make a world of difference in the way you feel and, in particular, how stressed you feel. Recent studies show that exercise has a remarkable ability to smooth moods—calming you down when you're stressed or tense or boosting your spirits when you're feeling depressed. Exercise can also improve your self-confidence and even help you think better and be more creative.

Here are some of the ways that exercise can help lift your emotions and improve your outlook on life:

Help for anxiety. Feelings of tension and anxiety often accompany depression. According to a recent analysis of 159 studies on exercise's impact on anxiety, exercise can reduce these feelings as effectively as traditional relaxation techniques such as meditation. The emotional high from a single workout can last at least several hours afterward and possibly much longer.

Even more significantly, regular exercise has been found to curb anxiety even after the glow from a workout has faded, especially in people suffering from chronic anxiety. Aerobic exercise improves mood and eases stress better than non-aerobic exercises such as strength training and stretching exercises.

But if you think that the exercise you do must be strenuous to improve your mood, you're wrong: At least four clinical trials have now shown that light to moderate exercise works as well as vigorous exercise to relieve stress and anxiety. In one of those trials, mild workouts actually eased anxiety faster.

In this study, Indiana University researchers asked 15 volunteers to perform leg exercises for 20-minute sessions at varying levels of intensity. Questionnaires showed equal drops in anxiety after a mild, moderate, or vigorous workout. But after a mild or moderate workout, anxiety dropped within just five minutes and stayed low until the researchers stopped measuring two hours later. But with the vigorous workout, anxiety levels didn't fall until an hour after the workout ended—perhaps because strenuous exercise initially is more stressful than calming.

Defeating depression. Studies consistently show that people who are physically active are less depressed than inactive people. But is that because exercise actually reduces depression or merely because depressed people don't feel like exercising? To find out which is the case, 10 studies have assigned depressed volunteers either to exercise, to receive some other treatment, or just to remain inactive. In all 10 studies, exercise was found to significantly reduce mild to moderate depression. In addition, three of the studies compared exercise to psychotherapy and found that exercise was at least as effective.

Any kind of exercise—strenuous or mild, rhythmic or nonrhythmic—seems to lift depression, perhaps because of a number of physiological effects on the body. Animal studies show that physical activity increases brain levels of key neurotransmitters that have a major influence on mood, including noradrenaline, serotonin, and dopamine. Exercise also increases the flow of oxygen-rich blood to the brain and increases levels of morphinelike chemicals in the body—the endorphins—that can have a positive effect on mood. And it works not only for physically healthy people but also for people with arthritis and other chronic conditions.

In women, regular exercise may even help prevent depression from developing in the first place. Researchers at the National Institute of Mental Health assessed the mood and habits of about 1,900 women and then reevaluated them eight years later. Among the women who weren't depressed at the start of the study, those who exercised at least occasionally were only half as likely to become depressed during the ensuing decade as those women who rarely or never exercised.

Improving self-esteem. People who are depressed often have negative feelings about themselves that may even include strong feelings of self-loathing. If you tend to have a poor self-image, exercise can help you feel better about yourself and give you more confidence that you can handle life's challenges.

The positive effect of exercise on self-image has been shown by clinical trials that have tested the link between exercise and what's known as "self-efficacy"—the confidence that you can master life's challenges. All six of the studies that have looked at the connection between exercise and self-efficacy have found that exercise boosts this type of confidence. Other studies have found that exercise raises self-esteem—especially when it comes to feelings about fitness and overall appearance.

If it does nothing else, a workout can provide a brief emotional lift. Even a brisk walk lasting 10 minutes is enough to make you feel more relaxed and energetic, and regular workouts produce more lasting improvements. For example, researchers at the University of Washington assigned 121 older volunteers either to a lengthy program of walking and running or to a control group that didn't exercise. All participants were evaluated after one year, and the exercisers felt substantially better—less anxious, less lonely, more satisfied with life, and less worried about growing old—than the inactive group did.

TAKING THE PLUNGE

Three types of exercises—aerobic, stretching, and strengthening—should be included in a well-rounded exercise regimen. The federal government's exercise prescription calls for about 30 minutes a day of mild to moderate exercise most days of the week, preferably every day. The workout can be continuous or accumulated in chunks throughout the day.

Aerobic exercise. Any exercise that raises your heart rate is an aerobic exercise, including walking. These exercises increase your overall fitness by training your heart and lungs to deliver oxygen more efficiently to the working muscles of the body. Regular aerobic exercise reduces the risk of several important killers, including high blood pressure, coronary heart disease, diabetes, and possibly cancer. In addition, aerobic exercise often serves as strengthening or stretching exercise for the joints. Swimming, for example, is both an excellent aerobic exercise and ideal for stretching. Walking and jogging are aerobic and also help build strength in leg and thigh muscles.

Stretching. These exercises move your joints through their full range of motion and, gently, even a bit further. And when you stretch a muscle slightly beyond its normal length, it gradually adapts to its new length, improving muscle elasticity as well as joint flexibility. A good stretching routine is an excellent way to relax and to reduce stress—as exemplified by yoga, which both increases flexibility and enhances a person's feelings of well-being.

Strength training. Increasingly, studies are showing that strength-training exercises—lifting weights, pulling against the resistance of stretchable latex bands, or working out on Nautilus or other strength-training equipment—should be an integral part of an exercise regimen. It can restore the muscle strength we lose as we age, help fend off weight gain, improve balance and mobility, help strengthen bones, and reduce the risk of heart attack and diabetes in ways that aerobic exercise doesn't. And in a recent study, strength training was shown to reduce depression in older people, who often can't tolerate the side effects of antidepressants.

It's important to realize that there *are* things you can do to help lift your depression. These actions can range from seeking the help of a mental health professional to giving up smoking to engaging in a strength-training program. In the next chapter, we move from the mind to the body, with a look at some of the surprising benefits to physical health that St. John's wort can offer.

❧ CHAPTER 10 ❧

Antibiotic, Anti-Inflammatory, and Other Benefits of St. John's Wort

For more than 2,000 years, herbal healers have valued St. John's wort at least as much for its ability to heal the body as for its aid to the psyche. One of the most ancient uses of St. John's wort—as a "vulnerary," or wound-healing agent—persists to this day. The herb has also been recommended for use against snakebite, as a diuretic, to clear up infections, reduce inflammation, and for treating painful conditions such as sciatica and hip pain.

These and other bodily benefits of St. John's wort have only recently been looked at scientifically. In many cases, the acumen of the ancient herbal healers has been borne out. In this chapter, we'll take a look at some of the ways that St. John's wort can help heal the body.

WOUND HEALING

St. John's wort has long been recommended for its wound-healing abilities. More than 300 years ago, in 1663, the herbalist Gerard wrote that St. John's wort was unequaled as a balm for wounds, bites, burns, and ulcerations. And indeed, the ability of St. John's wort to heal wounds is one of the herb's most thoroughly documented benefits.

In 1975, researchers prepared a St. John's wort burn ointment by combining five grams of fresh St. John's wort flowers with 100 grams of olive oil and letting the mixture sit at room temperature for 10 days. They then used the ointment on first-, second-, and third-degree burns.

First-degree burns that were treated with the ointment healed within 48 hours. Second- and third-degree burns were found to heal at least three times as fast as burns that were treated with conventional burn treatments; in addition, the St. John's wort ointment inhibited the formation of keloids—protruding scars caused by the continuing production of scar tissue long after healing would usually be complete.

The usefulness of St. John's wort ointment is not limited to wound healing. For example, Native Americans have long used it as a salve for treating snakebite. And herbal healers in various parts of the world have recommended St. John's wort as a treatment for hemorrhoids, bruises, sprains, and contusions.

In addition to healing wounds when applied as an ointment, St. John's wort may also help against wounds when taken internally. In a 1991 study, researchers studied the wound-healing properties of an orally administered tincture of St. John's wort. They compared it with calendula, another widely used wound-healing herb, which was used topically. The oral St. John's wort preparation was found to be more effective in healing wounds than the topically applied calendula.

ANTIBACTERIAL POWER

The ability of St. John's wort to heal wounds may stem partly from its ability to act as a natural antibiotic—an effect that is probably due to several of the herb's components. Two of the chemicals isolated from St. John's wort were found to have an antibacterial effect that was more potent than the effect of the antibiotic sulfonilamide. In addition, antibacterial activity is attributed to the essential oil in St. John's wort and to several groups of chemicals present in the herb—the tannins, the phloroglucinols, and the flavonoids.

Studies have shown that an alcohol extract of St. John's wort exhibits not only potent antibacterial activity but some antifungal activity as well. An alcohol extract was also found to be effective against gram-positive bacteria, and the tannins and flavonoids extracted from the herb were able to inactivate E. coli bacteria even when they were present in very dilute amounts. E. coli is the most common cause of urinary tract infections, and Russian researchers recently recommended extracts of St. John's wort as a possible way to prevent these infections from occurring. Consult your doctor before embarking on a treatment plan that uses St. John's wort for its antibiotic properties.

A POTENT VIRUS KILLER

The presence of St. John's wort is not always viewed with pleasure. In fact, as described earlier, farmers and ranchers in the western United States often regard St. John's wort as a noxious weed because cattle that graze on large amounts of St. John's wort and then stand in sunlight may develop severe sunburn. The chemical in the herb responsible for this photosensitizing effect is hypericin, a red pigment that is found almost exclusively in St. John's wort. When St. John's wort is swallowed, the hypericin is absorbed by the body's tissues, including the skin; when skin cells are exposed to light, hypericin reacts with the light to form chemicals that are toxic to the cells. But ironically, this reaction that can be fatal to cows could prove lifesaving to humans.

St. John's wort has a proven ability to inactivate viruses, and photosensitization seems to account for the herb's virus-killing ability. Studies have shown that two of the main components of St.

John's wort—hypericin and pseudohypericin—
can effectively inactivate so-called encapsulated
viruses, including herpes simplex type 1 (the cause
of recurrent cold sores) as well as two viruses that
have a major impact on public health: herpes simplex type 2 (the cause of genital herpes) and HIV,
the virus that causes AIDS.

Hypericin, the main active ingredient in St.
John's wort, seems to be the key antiviral ingredient. But hypericin is found at relatively low levels in St. John's wort—far less than one percent of
the total herb. As a result, most of the antiviral
studies involving St. John's wort have used a pu-
rified synthetic version of hypericin, allowing researchers to give much higher doses of hypericin
than would be possible if they had to rely on extracts of the herb.

The interest in St. John's wort as a treatment for
AIDS was sparked by a 1988 report in the prestigious Proceedings of the National Academy of Sciences, which described studies in which hypericin
was tested against the Friend leukemia virus, a
mouse virus that strongly resembles HIV.

The researchers found they could completely
prevent the rapid onset of disease and death in the
mice by giving them a single small dose of hypericin within a day after infecting them with the
Friend leukemia virus. Their conclusion: hypericin had "dramatic" antiviral activity and little toxicity at effective doses.

Success of the mouse studies led to a federally
sponsored clinical trial, beginning in 1991, in

which hypericin was tested on AIDS patients at three U.S. medical centers. Patients in the study were given high doses of synthetic hypericin, administered intravenously twice a week.

The study showed that the majority of the AIDS patients improved on the hypericin. But unfortunately, the patients themselves were affected by light exposure after they'd taken the high doses of hypericin; several of them had to withdraw from the study after experiencing phototoxicity reactions that included a tingling or burning sensation in the skin.

These side effects limited the amount of hypericin that the researchers could administer, preventing them from using a dose high enough that might have shown an effect against HIV. Although clinical trials of hypericin have now been abandoned, some researchers haven't given up on hypericin as an AIDS therapy. They remain hopeful that it may yet play a role in treating AIDS, perhaps as one component of a "cocktail" of drugs. (The levels of hypericin that caused the side effects in the AIDS patients were many times higher than the amount present in standard, antidepressant doses of St. John's wort extracts.)

Some of the same researchers involved in testing hypericin against HIV infections are also studying its usefulness in preventing the spread of viruses through blood transfusions. In these studies, hypericin was added to units of blood that had purposely been contaminated with HIV. When the blood was then illuminated with a fluorescent light for one hour, the researchers later found that all the contaminating viruses in the blood had been inactivated.

One type of virus that has proven resistant to any type of therapy is hepatitis C, which causes more than 150,000 new cases of hepatitis each year in the United States. Hypericin has shown promise against hepatitis C and, in a clinical trial now under way at two medical centers in New York City, it is being tried as a treatment on patients who have chronic hepatitis C.

Warts, which are also caused be virus infections, have resisted most treatment efforts short of surgery to excise them or burn them off. In 1997, a study was begun in which synthetic hypericin is being used to treat warts and other virus-caused skin diseases. Results of this study should be available by 1999.

A PROMISING CANCER FIGHTER

St. John's wort's photosensitizing ability may also make it a useful treatment against several types of cancer. In this type of treatment, known as photodynamic therapy, a photosensitizing agent is administered and becomes absorbed into a patient's tissues; the tissues are then exposed to a light source.

In recent laboratory studies, hypericin from St. John's wort has shown a potent effect against gliomas, the most common type of brain cancer and one that often proves fatal. Hypericin's anti-glioma impact reportedly equals or even exceeds that of tamoxifen, one of the most widely used cancer chemotherapy drugs. The gliomas responded to hypericin even in the absence of light; but exposure to visible light increased the killing effect by nearly 15 percent.

In welcome contrast to the HIV studies, hypericin seems to achieve its effect against tumors at doses low enough so that phototoxicity would probably not be a problem for patients. Currently a small clinical trial is underway in North Dakota in which a synthetic form of hypericin is being used to treat severely ill patients whose gliomas have not responded to any other treatment.

Melanoma is another often-deadly type of cancer that may respond to St. John's wort. Researchers at UCLA are experimenting with hypericin as a potential treatment for melanoma as well as squamous cell carcinoma, the most common type of skin cancer.

In recent studies, UCLA researchers implanted human cancer tissue under the skin of laboratory animals, so that the tissue would develop into tumors. The animals then ate food that contained hypericin. When the researchers exposed the animals to a laser light, they observed a tumor-destroying effect that was far greater than the effect produced by either the hypericin or the laser light alone. Dr. Daniel Castro, the UCLA researcher who is leading the hypericin research, said that hypericin "appears to be very promising" as a treatment for cancer.

IMPROVED BLOOD FLOW

St. John's wort may also have beneficial effects on the heart, according to recent research. In a study involving guinea pigs, researchers found that chemicals known as procyanidins, isolated from St. John's wort, enhanced the flow of blood through coronary arteries. The same researchers then tested procyanidins on pigs' hearts. They found that the St. John's wort chemicals effectively blocked the action of histamine and prostaglandin F, two chemicals known for their ability to cause arteries to constrict.

MELATONIN STIMULATOR

You've probably heard the recent buzz about melatonin, the hormone secreted by the pineal gland that has been found to play several crucial roles in the body. Melatonin supplements have been reported to help in treating jet lag, insomnia, stress, and depression and may also be useful in combating the degenerative effects of aging. Now there is evidence that St. John's wort may offer a "natural" way to raise melatonin levels.

In a recent study, researchers found that a commercial St. John's wort preparation caused a significant rise in nighttime melatonin levels after three weeks of daily use. Since nighttime is the optimal time for taking melatonin to relieve insomnia, this study suggests that St. John's wort's proven ability to improve sleep may be due to its ability to increase melatonin levels. Furthermore, melatonin has been shown to raise brain levels of serotonin, the neurotransmitter whose brain levels are also boosted by Prozac and similar antidepressants. Therefore, this ability of St. John's wort to stimulate melatonin production could partly explain why this herb has proven so effective in treating depression.

ANTI-INFLAMMATORY EFFECT

Whether applied topically or taken orally, St. John's wort can help to relieve the pain and inflammation caused by irritated nerves—presumably the reason that the herb has long been used as a treatment for sciatica (pain that radiates from the sciatic nerve, the large nerve that runs down the back of the thigh). St. John's wort appears to work by inhibiting the release of chemicals that are known to trigger inflammation.

Studies have suggested that St. John's wort can relieve the pain and inflammation following tooth extraction; the pain and inflammation from shingles (herpes zoster); the chronic nerve pain resulting from fractures, spinal injuries, musculoskeletal trauma and surgical trauma; and the burning or tingling pain as well as the twitching or spasm that can result from a traumatic injury.

ST. JOHN'S WORT FOR WEIGHT LOSS?

If an herb is known by the company it keeps then St. John's wort is in danger of having its enviable reputation tarnished. The reason: Some manufacturers are now concocting weight-loss products by combining St. John's wort with metabolism-stimulating drugs. Ephedra, the herbal stimulant also known as ma huang that is used in some of these products, has been linked to illnesses and deaths.

These combination weight-loss products are sold as "herbal fen-phen" or under similar names. They began appearing in September 1997, shortly after the FDA requested the recall of the two prescription drugs (fenfluramine and dexfenfluramine) that provided the "fen" portion of the *real* fen/phen weight-loss combination. (Phentermine, the "phen" half of the combo, remains available.) The two drugs were withdrawn because of reports that they could damage heart valves in up to 30 percent of people who took them. Now that the prescription weight-loss drugs are no longer available, marketers are touting herbal fen/phen products as "safer, more natural" alternatives. But that's a dubious claim, particularly for herbal combos that contain ephedra.

Ephedra's active ingredients (ephedrine, pseudoephedrine, and norpseudoephedrine) are known as ephedrine alkaloids—amphetaminelike compounds that can have powerful stimulant effects on the nervous system and heart. Since 1994, the FDA has received more than 800 reports of illnesses—including at least 17 deaths—involving people who have taken ma huang and other products containing ephedrine alkaloids. Most cases involved healthy adults who took the products for weight control or to increase energy. In June 1997, the FDA issued a proposal that would drastically reduce the amount of ephedrine alkaloids that would be allowed in dietary supplements.

St. John's wort is included in herbal fen/phen products in order to boost serotonin levels in the brain. But as noted in Chapter Five, it's not yet clear which of the brain's neurotransmitters are affected by St. John's wort. And an FDA spokeswoman said that the agency knew of "no information that St. John's wort is effective in weight loss." The best advice regarding herbal fen/phen products: Avoid them.

Although St. John's wort won't help you lose weight, this chapter shows that it offers a surprising number of other benefits for maintaining physical health. Indeed, it would be difficult to find another product that heals wounds, kills bacteria and viruses, holds promise for treating cancer, improves blood flow to the heart, and reduces inflammation.

If you've arrived at this point in the book and want to know more about what St. John's wort can offer, the next chapter may be just what the doctor ordered. It addresses questions that may have occurred to you, especially if you're thinking seriously of giving St. John's wort a try.

❖ CHAPTER 11 ❖

Questions and Answers About St. John's Wort

In this chapter, we answer some of the questions that may have arisen as you've been reading about St. John's wort and its usefulness in treating problems both mental and physical.

Q: *How long do I have to take St. John's wort before I start to feel its effects?*
A: As is the case with synthetic antidepressants, people must usually take St. John's wort for between two and six weeks before they notice a change in their mood. Just why there is such a time lag is one of the great unsolved mysteries of psychopharmacology. Synthetic antidepressants (and presumably St. John's wort as well) increase levels of neurotransmitters almost immediately, yet depressions typically do not lift until at least two weeks after treatment has begun.

One possible explanation: Antidepressants work by increasing the levels of neurotransmitter molecules in the gap between nerve cells; in turn, these neurotransmitters signal the adjacent nerve cell by fitting onto receptor molecules on their surface. In a sense, the neurotransmitters can be envisioned as "keys" that fit into the receptor "ignitions" on adjacent cells. But even while antidepressants may help to produce more of these neurotransmitter "keys," they may at the same time gum up the receptors into which those keys fit. These clogged-up receptor "ignitions" remain inaccessible, at least temporarily, to the neurotransmitter "keys"—which could explain the time lag between when treatment starts and when it takes effect.

The general rule of antidepressant therapy is this: If an antidepressant hasn't helped you after you've taken it for eight weeks, you should be switched to another one that may work better. Similarly, if you still feel depressed after taking St. John's wort for eight weeks, you should consult your doctor. You may need to take a synthetic antidepressant.

Q: *Does St. John's wort relieve depression as rapidly as the synthetic antidepressants such as Prozac?*
A: It's a little slower, but it does catch up. The clinical studies that have compared St. John's wort and standard antidepressants have generally lasted four to six weeks; by the end of that time, both medications have generally been found

equally effective, with about 60 percent of patients in each group experiencing significant improvement in their mood. But weekly evaluation of patients throughout some of these studies has shown that it generally takes St. John's wort a longer time to reach maximum effectiveness than it does for the synthetic antidepressants.

Q: *Once I find that St. John's wort has improved my mood, how long should I continue to take it?*
A: It's difficult to say. Most of the clinical studies on St. John's wort have lasted from four to six weeks—long enough to show that most depressed people who take the herb will successfully respond to it within that time span. And once your mood lifts, there's no rule that says you have to continue taking the herb.

Just as people with a middle-ear infection don't need to take an antibiotic for months on end after their infection has cleared up, depressed people who've take St. John's wort for awhile need not take it indefinitely. Furthermore, we know of no reports of side effects that have occurred when people have abruptly halted their St. John's wort regimen, although it may be wiser to taper off gradually.

As yet, studies in which people are "maintained" on St. John's wort simply haven't been done (although, as described in Chapter Five, the National Institutes of Health is sponsoring a major clinical study that will address that issue).

It's possible that longer-term use of St. John's

wort will reveal that side effects occur that haven't been discovered in the four- to six-week studies carried out up until now. That seems unlikely, since the herb has an enviable safety record that extends from centuries ago to the present day, with millions of people now taking St. John's wort and scarcely any problems reported. But to be on the safe side, you should probably consult your doctor if you're planning to use St. John's wort for several months.

Q: *My 70-year-old father has been feeling down ever since his retirement two years ago. Should I suggest that he look into taking St. John's wort?*
A: Absolutely. For people 60 and older, St. John's wort holds particular appeal compared with the standard antidepressants. Studies suggest that people over 60 are more sensitive than younger people to synthetic antidepressants. This means they can usually be treated with lower doses, but also that they're at greater risk for developing adverse effects from these drugs.

St. John's wort, on the other hand, appears to be quite safe for adults of all ages. As discussed more fully in Chapter Five, St. John's wort was the subject of a special issue of the *Journal of Geriatric Psychiatry and Neurology*, whose audience consists of doctors specializing in the psychological needs of the eldery. The journal's editor commented on the rarity of side effects caused by St. John's wort: "This benign side effect profile may make [St. John's wort] a particularly attractive choice for treating mild to moderate depression in our elderly patients."

Q: *I'd like to take something that would bump up my spirits a little, but I don't feel badly enough to be suffering from depression. Could I still benefit from taking St. John's wort.*
A: Definitely. The usefulness of St. John's wort in treating depression has only been established in the past 20 years through rigorously designed clinical studies. But long before the medical term "depression" was even coined—and going at least as far back as the ancient Greeks—folk healers have relied on St. John's wort as a tonic that can help soothe worry, anxiety, insomnia, and everything else that fit into the category of minor "nervous unrest."

If you feel depressed but perhaps not depressed enough to meet the definition of major depression (i.e., having five or more symptoms for a period of at least two weeks), you may have what is known as subclinical depression. Up until the past few years, people with subclinical depression weren't treated with antidepressants, since these drugs—with their high potential for causing serious side effects—were reserved for treating seriously depressed people.

But with the arrival of Prozac and other newer and less toxic antidepressants, doctors started prescribing antidepressants for their less severely depressed patients—and found that many of them were helped significantly. Since your depression is on the mild side, you may similarly find that St. John's wort provides the sort of boost for which you've been looking.

Although St. John's wort is sold as a dietary supplement and can be obtained without a prescription, it clearly acts like a drug in the body. And like any drug, St. John's wort shouldn't be taken casually. But when it comes to drugs that calm us down and elevate our moods, St. John's wort may well be the safest one available.

Q: *How much does it cost to take St. John's wort?*
A: Based on the products we've examined, it costs anywhere from 25 cents a day to one dollar a day. This estimate is based on the recommended daily doses of the most common dosage forms, capsules and tablets.

Q: *Is there any risk involved if I forget to take the recommended daily dose of St. John's wort?*
A: Probably not, as long as you miss only an occasional dose. For most St. John's wort products, the recommendation is to take several doses (typically three) per day. If you forget to take one dose—your afternoon capsule, for example—it is probably all right to take two capsules in the evening instead of the one that you would ordinarily take. But if you skip an entire day, it's probably not a good idea to compensate the next day by taking a double dose.

Although St. John's wort appears to cause fewer side effects than any other antidepressant, taking a double dose in one day might increase your risk of experiencing nausea, a rash, or one of the other usually minor side effects that have been attributed to St. John's wort. Of course, if you neglect to take St. John's wort or if you take it erratically, you lower the likelihood that it will be effective in improving your mood.

Q: *Is it all right to take St. John's wort if I'm trying to get pregnant?*
A: The standard recommendation for all medications, including antidepressants, is to avoid them if you are trying to get pregnant and during the first three months of pregnancy as well, in order to minimize the risk that the medication could harm the fetus in some way. Although no studies have been done on whether St. John's wort might pose a risk during pregnancy, information on antidepressants as a drug class is reassuring in this regard. No harmful effects have been observed in children whose fathers were taking antidepressants at the time of conception; similarly, harmful effects have not been found in children whose mothers were taking antidepressants shortly before conception occurred.

For women who are taking St. John's wort while they are nursing, it's quite possible that some of the chemicals in the herb will be present in their breast milk, since synthetic antidepressants have been found in breast milk as well. But the amounts of the synthetic antidepressants found in breast milk is quite low, so it's likely that chemicals from St. John's wort would similarly be present in very low concentrations. In view of the remarkable record of safety that St. John's wort has established, it's unlikely that a nursing baby would experience any adverse effects from the St. John's wort that its mother is taking. But to be on the safe side, it's best to consult your doctor about any medication, including St. John's wort, that you may be taking while trying to get pregnant, while pregnant, or when nursing.

Q: *What sort of change in mood should I experience while I am taking St. John's wort?*
A: In the many clinical studies in which St. John's wort has been studied, it has been found to elevate patients' mood—helping to dispel the blues and restoring a more normal emotional balance. And if you've been feeling anxious or have had trouble sleeping, St. John's wort should help to relieve these problems as well.

Q: *Claims about St. John's wort's effectiveness seem to be limited to saying that it helps in treating mild to moderate depression. Does that mean it doesn't work in cases of severe depression?*
A: Not much can be said about St. John's wort's effectiveness against severe depression because, up until now, it hasn't been tested against severe depression to any great extent. Whether in studies that have compared St. John's wort with a placebo or with a synthetic antidepressant, the patients involved in the study have mostly been people with mild to moderate depression.

One exception is a study described in Chapter Five, comparing St. John's wort with imipramine, a tricyclic antidepressant. This study involved 130 patients, 51 of whom were severely depressed at the start of the study. Overall, St. John's wort and imipramine were judged equally effective. But when patients were evaluated according to subgroup, St. John's wort proved significantly more effective than imipramine in treating the severely depressed patients.

One possible reason for this finding is that the dose of imipramine that was used in this study was somewhat on the low side. (The usual dose of imipramine for outpatients is 50 to 150 mg daily, and the dosage chosen for this study was 75 mg daily.) Nevertheless, at the conclusion of their study, the researchers stated: "In particular, there is still the question of . . . whether the general impression that [St. John's wort] extract is only suitable for mild or moderate depression needs to be corrected."

Clearly, what is needed are additional studies of St. John's wort in which severely depressed people are enrolled—and in which the herb is matched against a high enough dose of a synthetic drug to allow for a fair comparison. But until then, St. John's wort should be used for what it has been found so effective in treating: cases of mild to moderate depression.

Q: *Are there any foods that I should avoid if I'm taking St. John's wort?*
A: We know of no problems that have occurred

due to interactions between St. John's wort and any food. But you should be aware that some foods—and drinks—may blunt the effectiveness of St. John's wort. Drinking a lot of caffeinated coffee, for example, may cause anxiety, nervousness, and sleeplessness. And you should definitely try to minimize your use of alcohol while you're taking St. John's wort. Alcohol is a central nervous system depressant, and consuming alcohol while you're depressed or while you're taking St. John's wort is definitely not a good idea.

Q: *Is is okay for me to continue taking vitamins while I'm taking St. John's wort?*
A: By all means. In fact, certain vitamins may help to augment the antidepressant effect of St. John's wort. As discussed more fully in Chapter Eight, consuming adequate amounts of the B vitamins is especially important to mental health. For some women, taking oral contraceptives can cause a vitamin B_6 deficiency that can result in depression, and vitamin B_6 supplements can be important for treating this problem. Other B vitamin deficiencies can also be involved in depression. For example, a deficiency of vitamin B_{12} can cause depression along with pernicious anemia.

Q: *Is it safe to take St. John's wort if I'm also taking Prozac?*
A: According to experts we've spoken to, it's quite likely by now that hundreds of people have taken

St. John's wort and Prozac in combination, with no known reports of any problems. But to be on the safe side, it's probably best to take one or the other but not both. That's because, until recently, St. John's wort was thought to relieve depression in the same way that the monoamine oxidase inhibitor (MAOI) class of antidepressants do the job: by inactivating monamine oxidase, an enzyme that breaks down neurotransmitters in the brain.

Since taking an MAOI and Prozac in combination can cause severe and potentially fatal high blood pressure reactions, it was feared that the combination of St. John's wort and Prozac might also cause problems. But recent studies in animals have failed to show any MAOI activity when St. John's wort is given, although it remains possible that St. John's wort could still be exerting an MAOI effect in people. So for now, it's best to err on the side of caution and not take St. John's wort if you're also taking Prozac or similar-acting antidepressants such as Paxil and Zoloft.

Q: *Is one brand of St. John's wort known to be any better than others?*
A: So far, no studies have been done that have attempted to compare different brands of St. John's wort. In the clinical trials that have been done on St. John's wort—studies carried out primarily in Germany comparing the herb with either a placebo or one of the synthetic antidepressants—the brand most often used were the two brands of tablets that are manufactured by Lichtwer Pharma, a

German pharmaceutical company. For example, in a recent review of 25 controlled clinical studies that have used St. John's wort preparations, 13 of them used either Jarsin or Jarsin 300, the two Lichtwer Pharma brands of St. John's wort. Jarsin 300 is now the largest selling antidepressant in Germany. In 1997, Lichtwer Pharma began selling its Jarsin 300 in the U.S. under the name Kira, which is now available in drugstores and retail chain stores nationwide.

With some justification, the Kira box has the word "proven" stamped on it, and the product calls itself "the clinically proven hypericum formula (St. John's wort)." Nevertheless, many other products now on the market are essentially similar to Kira, i.e., their tablets or capsules contains 300 mg of dried herb extract made from the flowers and upper leaves of St. John's wort; and, like Kira, these other extracts have been standardized—tested and adjusted so that their concentration of hypericin is 0.3 percent.

Q: *When I buy a St. John's wort product, do I have any assurance that capsules, tablets, or liquids really do contain the ingredients that will help to lift my mood?*
A: Unfortunately, you don't. Compared with drugs, the manufacture of dietary supplements such as St. John's wort products receives little attention from the U.S. Food and Drug Administration. For example, FDA inspectors don't do what they do at the country's drug manufacturing fa-

cilities, which is to keep a close eye on quality control and check records to make sure that the proper ingredients are being used in every batch of the product. So with St. John's wort, for example, you just have to take the manufacturer's word that it really has standardized its extract so that the concentration of hypericin is 0.3 percent.

Nevertheless, some supplement makers have their own production and quality control standards that rival those used by the pharmaceutical companies. Some firms, for example, test every batch of a supplement they make, to assure that products are free from impurities and that the products contain the correct amounts of the active ingredients.

If you're curious about the way a St. John's wort product is made, write or call the manufacturer and ask for information on their testing and other quality control procedures. (The table beginning on page 138 lists the phone numbers for manufacturers of most of the St. John's wort products listed.) In particular, you should ask the company if it meets FDA standards for making food products. Companies that devote a lot of attention to quality are usually happy to tell you how their products are made.

Q: *My doctor has given me the go-ahead to take St. John's wort for my depressed mood, but he says that I'll have to pay for it out of my own pocket. Is he right?*
A: Unfortunately, yes. Since St. John's wort is clas-

sified in the U.S. as a dietary supplement and not as a drug, it is not covered by most health insurance policies.

Q: *My health food store carries a product in which St. John's wort is combined with several other herbs including valerian root and kava kava root. Is there any advantage to taking this sort of combination product?*
A: Not really, and there could be some disadvantages to taking St. John's wort as part of an herbal complex. Over the many centuries in which it has been used, St. John's wort has established an impressive record for effectiveness as well as safety. And the clinical studies of the past decade have provided further confirmation that this herb is remarkably safe to use. But just as prescription drugs are known to interact with each other to cause potentially dangerous side effects, taking St. John's wort along with other herbs could also increase your chances of experiencing toxic reactions. To gain the maximum benefit from St. John's wort with the least risk of side effects, you should stick with single-ingredient preparations of the herb.

Q: *I tried taking a standard antidepressant the last time I felt depressed and really didn't experience any improvement. Is there any reason to think that St. John's wort will work any better for me?*
A: St. John's wort may be *particularly* useful for you and other people who have tried synthetic

medications and haven't been helped by them. That's because St. John's wort seems to work *differently* against depression than today's standard antidepressants, whose effects are pretty much limited to bolstering brain levels of three neurotransmitters—serotonin, dopamine, and norepinephrine.

Since not everyone is helped by these drugs and the changes in neurotransmitter levels that they bring about, it's entirely possible that "nonresponders" like yourself could benefit from the physiological changes produced by St. John's wort. The fact that researchers still don't know how St. John's wort alleviates depression shouldn't be a cause for concern: Some 25 clinical studies—plus the actual experience of millions of people who've taken St. John's wort—show that this is an effective as well as remarkably safe medicinal herb that is much less likely to cause side effects than any of the standard antidepressant drugs.

❖ CHAPTER 12 ❖

Resources

GENERAL RESOURCES FOR DEPRESSION

The National Institute of Mental Health's Depression Awareness, Recognition and Treatment Program (D/ART) offers several free booklets that may be useful for people suffering from depression. They include "Plain Talk About Depression," "Depressive Illnesses: Treatments Bring New Hope," and "Medications," which reviews the different types of antidepressant medications and their side effects. You can order them by calling 800-421-4211.

The American Psychiatric Association's Division of Public Affairs (202-682-6220) in Washington, D.C., will provide you with referrals to psychiatrists in your area who specialize in treating depression.

The National Depressive and Manic-Depressive
Association
730 Franklin St., Suite 501
Chicago, IL 60610
800-826-3632
This organization distributes information on depression and bipolar illness (manic depression)
and also offers referrals to support groups in your
area.

The National Foundation for Depressive Illness
P.O. Box 2257
New York, NY 10116
800-239-1263
http://www.depression.org
This organization can provide you with physician
referrals, help in finding support groups in your
area, and information about depression.

National Mental Health Association
1021 Prince St.
Alexandria, VA 22314-2971
800-969-NMHA (6642)
Provides referrals to mental health providers and
free information on more than 200 mental health
topics.

National Alliance for the Mentally Ill
200 North Glebe Rd., Suite 1015
Arlington, VA 22203-3754
800-950-NAMI (6264)

Provides written material on a wide variety of mental illnesses.

The Anxiety Disorders Association of America
6000 Executive Blvd., Suite 513
Rockville, Md. 20852
301-231-9350
Provides information on anxiety disorders and a list of specialists in your area; enclose a check for $3 with your request.

HERBAL RESOURCES

Interested in learning more about medicinal herbs? A new bimonthly magazine, *Herbs for Health*, provides a good introduction to the field. To obtain a year's subscription costing $24, call 888-844-3727.

If you're really serious about herbs, you'll want to subscribe to *HerbalGram*, the quarterly journal of the American Botanical Council and the Herb Research Foundation. This peer-reviewed scientific journal includes research reviews, book reviews, and regular discussions of legal issues pertaining to herbs. To subscribe to *HerbalGram* (four issues for $25), call 800-373-7105.

The Herb Research Foundation also offers information packets on 140 different herbs, including St. John's wort. To order, send a note requesting the St. John's wort packet along with a check for $7 to the foundation at 1007 Pearl St.,

Suite 200, Boulder, CO 80302. If you request it, the foundation will enclose a list of all 140 herbs for which information packets are available.

USING THE INTERNET

Having a computer and a modem allows you to go online for a wealth of information about depression and other health problems. A convenient way to access it all is by subscribing to one of the major online service providers such as America Online (AOL) or Prodigy.

AOL's Personal Empowerment Network (Keyword PEN) is a particularly useful resource. Once you're there, you'll see a list of health-related topics including "mental health issues and concerns." Click on that and you'll be presented with a menu offering additional information on mental health such as "stress and stress management," "mental health-related articles" and "depression: causes and concerns."

AOL's Personal Empowerment Network also lets you search the massive MEDLINE database for studies on depression or any other health topic; access software libraries that offer thousands of easy-to-download health-related resources that can run on Macintoshes or PC's; and enter chat rooms where people discuss a wide variety of health topics.

Another useful feature of AOL and the other online services: They give you access to the rest of the Internet, including sites on the World Wide Web and any one of several thousand newsgroups.

People read and post messages in newsgroups to discuss a variety of topics related to a central theme, such as depression. The newsgroups truly are forums for the free exchange of ideas, opinions, and questions. Whatever topic you're interested in, there's sure to be a newsgroup that covers it. Of the thousands of newsgroups accessible through AOL and other online services, several that are especially relevant to depression include:

alt.support.depression
soc.support.depression.crisis
soc.support.depression.family
soc.support.depression.seasonal
soc.support.depression.treatment

In a newsgroup you can read message "threads"—discussions that typically begin by someone asking a question, which in turn stimulates responses from others who are participating in the newsgroup. On a recent visit to the alt.support.depression newsgroup, we saw interesting message threads on dozens of issues including "exercise and depression," "SSRIs—long term use," "living with depression" and "side effects of Zoloft."

There are literally thousands of sites on the Internet's World Wide Web, but some that are particularly relevant to people interested in depression or herbs include the following:

Depression-related Web sites

Health World Online

http://www.healthy.net

This site calls itself "the home of self-managed care." It's a comprehensive and well-organized source of health information. Click on "diseases/conditions" on the home page and you get a long alphabetical listing that includes depression; click on depression and you'll find several useful articles on the subject. A click on "Health Clinic" will lead you to "Alternative & Complementary Therapies," where you can then home in on "Herbal Medicine."

Internet Mental Health

http://www.mentalhealth.com

This is a vast encyclopedia of mental health information designed by Canadian psychiatrist Phillip Long. Here you can find information on the 52 most common mental disorders and—for each one—a description, diagnostic and treatment information, and research findings. Internet Mental Health also makes available recent magazine articles on mental health and offers "links" to other useful mental health sites on the World Wide Web.

Mental Health Net

http://www.cmhc.com

A site that provides information on the treatment of depression as well as links to other depression-related Web sites.

Dr. Ivan's Depression Central
http://www. psycom.net/depression.central.html
A central clearinghouse for information on and treatment of many types of depressive disorders including major depression, manic depression (bipolar disorder), and dysthymia.

HealthGuide
http://www.healthguide.com
Offers clearly written, basic information on health topics of all kinds including mental, family, and physical health. Click on "depression" under "Diagnoses" and then obtain a variety of information on depression including "why depression occurs," "types of depression," and "treatment."

Herb-related Web sites
http://www.hypericum.com
A site devoted entirely to St. John's wort. Lists products and prices and offers useful information and advice for people interested in taking St. John's wort products.

http://www.botanical.com
Sponsored by several herb companies, this site offers reviews of herb books and practical information on topics such as "how to make incense." Also contains an interesting description of St. John's wort from *A Modern Herbal*, the classic 1931 text written by Mrs. M. Grieve.

Natural Health and Longevity World Wide Web
Resource Center
http://www.all-natural.com
Contains a useful herb reference library.

Henriette's Herbal Homepage
http://sunsite.unc.edu/herbmed
Offers a large amount of herbal information on
herbal topics including medicinal and culinary
herbs, answers to frequently asked questions
about herbs, and pictures of different herbs.

LARRY KATZENSTEIN is the former medical editor of *American Health* magazine and served for twelve years as a health writer at *Consumer Reports*. He has earned national recognition for his medical writing, including the New York Newspaper Guild's Page One Award for Excellence in Journalism, the American College of Allergy and Immunology Media Award, and the William Harvey Award for Journalistic Achievement in Hypertension.